# Tools and Methods of Gene Therapy

# Tools and Methods of Gene Therapy

Edited by **Harvey Summers**

FOSTER
ACADEMICS

New Jersey

Published by Foster Academics,
61 Van Reypen Street,
Jersey City, NJ 07306, USA
www.fosteracademics.com

**Tools and Methods of Gene Therapy**
Edited by Harvey Summers

© 2015 Foster Academics

International Standard Book Number: 978-1-63242-406-8 (Hardback)

# Contents

# Preface

The main aim of this book is to educate learners and enhance their research focus by presenting diverse topics covering this vast field. This is an advanced book which compiles significant studies by distinguished experts in the area of analysis. This book addresses successive solutions to the challenges arising in the area of application, along with it; the book provides scope for future developments.

The state-of-the-art information regarding gene therapy has been included in this book. Gene Therapy as a field has gained its due regard after all these years of poor outcomes. Issues in the past which were troubling scientists and practitioners are now being easily resolved. The growth of secure and effective gene transfer and development in the field of cell therapy has now brought new ways to deal with varied diseases. The book aims at compiling information from different resources about various applications and inherited diseases, discussing important topics such as gene therapy for retinitis pigmentosa, primary immunodeficiencies, molecular therapy for lysosomal storage diseases, and clinical and translational challenges in gene therapy of cardiovascular diseases.

It was a great honour to edit this book, though there were challenges, as it involved a lot of communication and networking between me and the editorial team. However, the end result was this all-inclusive book covering diverse themes in the field.

Finally, it is important to acknowledge the efforts of the contributors for their excellent chapters, through which a wide variety of issues have been addressed. I would also like to thank my colleagues for their valuable feedback during the making of this book.

**Editor**

# Introduction

# Non-Viral Delivery Systems in Gene Therapy

Alicia Rodríguez Gascón,
Ana del Pozo-Rodríguez and María Ángeles Solinís

Additional information is available at the end of the chapter

## 1. Introduction

Recent advances in molecular biology combined with the culmination of the Human Genome Project [1] have provided a genetic understanding of cellular processes and disease pathogenesis; numerous genes involved in disease and cellular processes have been identified as targets for therapeutic approaches. In addition, the development of high-throughput screening techniques (e.g., cDNA microarrays, differential display and database meaning) may drastically increase the rate at which these targets are identified [2,3]. Over the past years there has been a remarkable expansion of both the number of human genes directly associated with disease states and the number of vector systems available to express those genes for therapeutic purposes. However, the development of novel therapeutic strategies using these targets is dependent on the ability to manipulate the expression of these target genes in the desired cell population. In this chapter we explain the concept and aim of gene therapy, the different gene delivery systems and therapeutic strategies, how genes are delivered and how they reach the target.

## 2. Aim and concept of gene therapy with non-viral vectors

A gene therapy medicinal product is a biological product which has the following characteristics: (a) it contains an active substance which contains or consists of a recombinant nucleic acid used in administered to human beings with a view to regulating, repairing, replacing, adding or deleting a genetic sequence; (b) its therapeutic, prophylactic or diagnostic effect relates directly to the recombinant nucleic acid sequence it contains, or to the product of genetic expression of this sequence [4].

The most important, and most difficult, challenge in gene therapy is the issue of delivery. The tools used to achieve gene modification are called gene therapy vectors and they are the "key" for an efficient and safe strategy. Therefore, there is a need for a delivery system, which must first overcome the extracellular barriers (such as avoiding particle clearance mechanisms, targeting specific cells or tissues and protecting the nucleic acid from degradation) and, subsequently, the cellular barriers (cellular uptake, endosomal escape, nuclear entry and nucleic release) [5]. An ideal gene delivery vector should be effective, specific, long lasting and safe.

Gene therapy has long been regarded a promising treatment for many diseases, including inherited through a genetic disorder (such as hemophilia, human severe combined immunodeficiency, cystic fibrosis, etc) or acquired (such as AIDS or cancer). Figures 1 and 2 show the indications addressed and the gene types transferred in gene therapy clinical trials, respectively [6].

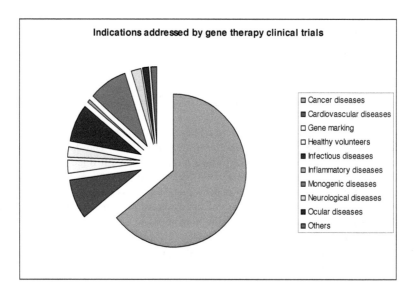

**Figure 1.** Indications addressed by gene therapy clinical trials (adapted from http://www.wiley.co.k/genmed/clinical).

Gene delivery systems include viral vectors and non-viral vectors. Viral vectors are the most effective, but their application is limited by their immunogenicity, oncogenicity and the small size of the DNA they can transport. Non-viral vectors are safer, of low cost, more reproducible and do not present DNA size limit. The main limitation of non-viral systems is their low transfection efficiency, although it has been improved by different strategies and the efforts are still ongoing [6]; actually, advances of non-viral delivery have lead to an increased number of products entering into clinical trials. However, viral vector has dominated the clinical trials in gene therapy for its relatively high delivery efficiency. Figure 3 shows the proportion of vector systems currently in human trials [7].

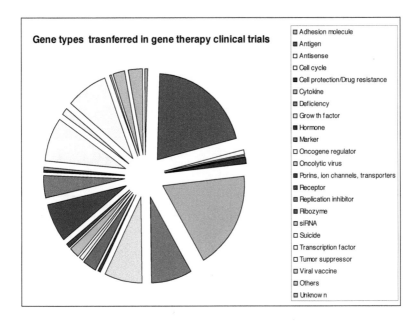

**Figure 2.** Gene types transferred in gene therapy clinical trials (adapted from http://www.wiley.co.k/genmed/clinical).

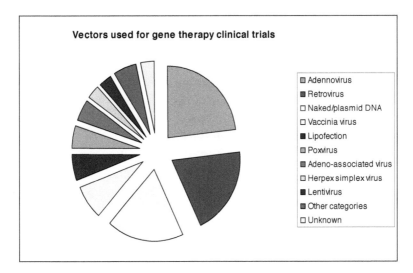

**Figure 3.** Vector systems used in gene therapy clinical trials (adapted from http://www.wiley.co.k/genmed/clinical).

## 3. Non-viral methods for transfection

Currently, three categories of non-viral systems are available:

• Inorganic particles

• Synthetic or natural biodegradable particles

• Physical methods

Table 1 summarizes the most utilized non-viral vectors.

| Category | System for gene delivery |
|---|---|
| Inorganic particles | Calcium phosphate |
|  | Silica |
|  | Gold |
|  | Magnetic |
| Synthetic or natural biodegradable particles | 1. Polymeric-based non-viral vectors: |
|  | Poly(lactic-co-glycolic acid) (PLGA) |
|  | Poly lactic acid (PLA) |
|  | Poly(ethylene imine) (PEI) |
|  | Chitosan |
|  | Dendrimers |
|  | Polymethacrylates |
|  | 2. Cationic lipid-based non-viral vectors: |
|  | Cationic liposomes |
|  | Cationic emulsions |
|  | Solid lipid nanoparticles |
|  | 3. Peptide-based non-viral vectors: |
|  | Poly-L-lysine |
|  | Other peptides to functionalize other delivery systems: SAP, protamine |
| Physical methods | Needle injection |
|  | Balistic DNA injection |
|  | Electroporation |
|  | Sonoporation |
|  | Photoporation |
|  | Magnetofection |
|  | Hydroporation |

**Table 1.** Delivery systems for gene therapy.

## 3.1. Inorganic particles

Inorganic nanoparticles are nanostructures varying in size, shape and porosity, which can be engineered to evade the reticuloendothelial system or to protect an entrapped molecular payload from degradation or denaturation [8]. Calcium phosphate, silica, gold, and several magnetic compounds are the most studied [9-11]. Silica-coated nanoparticles are biocompatible structures that have been used for various biological applications including gene therapy due to its biocompatibility [8]. Mesoporous silica nanoparticles have shown gene transfection efficiency "in vitro" in glial cells [12]. Magnetic inorganic nanoparticles (such as $Fe_3O_4$, $MnO_2$) have been applied for cancer-targeted delivery of nucleic acids and simultaneous diagnosis via magnetic resonance imaging [13,14]. Silica nanotubes have been also studied as an efficient gene delivery and imaging agent [13].

Inorganic particles can be easily prepared and surface-functionalized. They exhibit good storage stability and are not subject to microbial attack [13]. Bhattarai et al. [15] modified mesoporous silica nanoparticles with poly(ethylene glycol) and methacrylate derivatives and used them to deliver DNA or small interfering RNA (siRNA) "in vitro".

Gold nanoparticles have been lately investigated for gene therapy. They can be easily prepared, display low toxicity and the surface can be modified using various chemical techniques [16]. For instance, gold nanorods have been proposed to deliver nucleic acids to tumors [13]. They have strong absorption bands in the near-infrared region, and the absorbed light energy is then converted into heat by gold nanorods (photohermal effect). The near-infrared light can penetrate deeply into tissues; therefore, the surface of the gold could be modified with double-stranded DNA for controlled release [17]. After irradiation with near-infrared light, single stranded DNA is released due to thermal denaturation induced by the photothermal effect.

## 3.2. Synthetic or natural biodegradable particles

Synthetic or natural biocompatible particles may be composed by cationic polymers, cationic lipids or cationic peptides, and also the combination of these components [18-21]. The potential advantages of biodegradable carriers are their reduced toxicity (degradation leads to non-toxic products) and avoidance of accumulation of the polymer in the cells.

### 3.2.1. Polymer-based non-viral vectors

Cationic polymers condense DNA into small particles (polyplexes) and prevent DNA from degradation. Polymeric nanoparticles are the most commonly used type of nano-scale delivery systems. They are mostly spherical particles, in the size range of 1-1000 nm, carrying the nucleic acids of interest. DNA can be entrapped into the polymeric matrix or can be adsorbed or conjugated on the surface of the nanoparticles. Moreover, the degradation of the polymer can be used as a tool to release the plasmid DNA into the cytosol [22]. Table 1 shows several commonly used polymers used for gene delivery [16].

*3.2.1.1. Poly(lactic-co-glycolic acid) (PLGA) and poly lactic acid (PLA)*

Biodegradable polyesters, PLGA and PLA, are the most commonly used polymers for delivering drugs and biomolecules, including nucleic acids. They consist of units of lactic acid and glycolic acid connected through ester linkage. These biodegradable polymers undergo bulk hydrolysis thereby providing sustained delivery of the therapeutic agent. The degradation products, lactic acid and glycolic acid, are removed from the body through citric acid cycle. The release of therapeutic agent from these polymers occurs by diffusion and polymer degradation [16].

PLGA has a demonstrated FDA approved track record as a vehicle for drug and protein delivery [23,24]. Biodegradable PLA and PLGA particles are biocompatible and have the capacity to protect pDNA from nuclease degradation and increase pDNA stability [25,26].

PLGA particles typically less than 10 μm in size are efficiently phagocytosed by professional antigen presenting cells; therefore, they have significant potential for immunization applications [27,28]. For example, intramuscular immunization of p55 Gag plasmid adsorbed on PLGA/cetyl trimethyl ammonium bromide (CTAB) particles induced potent antibody and cytotoxic T lymphocyte responses. These particles showed a 250-fold increase in antibody response at higher DNA doses and more rapid and complete seroconversion, at the lower doses, compared to other adjuvants, including cationic liposomes [29].

The encapsulation efficiency of DNA in PLGA nanoparticles is not very high, and it depends on the molecular weight of the PLGA and on the hydrophobicity of the polymer, being the hydrophilic polymers those that provide higher loading efficiency [30]. To enhance the DNA loading, several strategies have been proposed. Kusonowiriyawong et al. [31] prepared cationic PLGA microparticles by dissolving cationic surfactants (like water insoluble stearylamine) in the organic solvent in which the PLGA was dissolved to prepare the microparticles. Another strategy was to reduce the negative charge of plasmid DNA by condensing it with poly(aminoacids) (like poly-L-lysine) before encapsulation in PLGA microparticles [32,33].

Normally, after an initial burst release, plasmid DNA release from PLGA particles occurs slowly during several days/weeks [22]. The degradation of the PLGA nanoparticles, through a bulk homogeneous hydrolytic process, determines the release of plasmid DNA. Consequently, it can be expected that the use of more hydrophilic PLGA not only improves the encapsulation efficiency of DNA, but also results in a faster release of plasmid DNA. Delivery of the plasmid DNA depends on the copolymer composition of the PLGA (lactic acid versus glycolic acid), molecular weight, particle size and morphology [22]. DNA release kinetics depends also on the plasmid incorporation technique; Pérea et al. [34] reported that nanoparticles prepared by the water-oil emulsion/diffusion technique released their content rapidly, whereas those obtained by the water-oil-emulsion method showed an initial burst followed by a slow release during at least 28 days.

PLGA and PLA based nanoparticles have also been used for "in vitro" RNAi delivery [35]. For instance, Hong et al. [36] have shown the effects of glucocorticoid receptor siRNA delivered using PLGA microparticles, on proliferation and differentiation capabilities of human mesenchymal stromal cells.

### 3.2.1.2. Chitosan

Chitosan [b(1-4)2-amino-2-deoxy-D-glucose] is a biodegradable polysaccharide copolymer of N-acetyl-D-glucosamine and D-glucosamine obtained by the alkaline deacetylation of chitin, which is a polysaccharide found in the exoskeleton of crustaceans of marine arthropods and insects [37]. Chitosans differ in the degree of N-acetylation (40 to 98%) and molecular weight (50 to 2000 kDa) [38]. As the only natural polysaccharide with a positive charge, chitosan has the following unique properties as carrier for gene therapy:

- it is potentially safe and non-toxic, both in experimental animals [39] and humans [40]

- it can be degraded into $H_2O$ and $CO_2$ in the body, which ensures its biosafety

- it has biocompatibility to the human body and does not elicit stimulation of the mucosa and the derma

- its cationic polyelectrolyte nature provides a strong electrostatic interaction with negatively charged DNA [41], and protects the DNA from nuclease degradation [42]

- the mucoadhesive property of chitosan potentially leads to a sustained interaction between the macromolecule being "delivered" and the membrane epithelia, promoting more efficient uptake [43]

- it has the ability to open intercellular tight junctions, facilitating its transport into the cells [44]

Currently, there is a commercial transfection reagent based on chitosan (Novafect, NovaMatrix, FMC, US), and many other prototypes are under development. Most of the chitosan-based nanocarriers for gene delivery have been based on direct complexation of chitosan and the nucleic acid [45], whereas in some instances additional polyelectrolytes, polymers and lipids have been used in order to form composite nanoparticles [46-49] or chitosan-coated hydrophobic nanocarriers.

Many studies using cell cultures have shown that pDNA-loaded chitosan nanocarriers are able to achieve high transfection levels in most cell lines [50]. Chitosan nanocarriers loaded with siRNA have provided gene suppression values similar to the commercial reagent lipofectamine [51,52,18,53].

Chitosan of low molecular weight is more efficient for transfection than chitosan with high molecular weight. This enhancement in transfection efficacy observed with low molecular weight chitosan can be attributed to the easier release of pDNA from the nanocarrier upon cell internalization. Moreover, the presence of free low molecular chitosan has been deemed to be very important for the endosomal escape of the nanocarriers [50]. Concerning deacetylation degree, its influence on transfection is not still clear. "In vitro" studies have shown that the best transfection is achieved with highly deacetylated chitosan [54,55]. However, "in

vivo", higher transfection was achieved after intramuscular administration of chitosan complexes with a low deacetylation degree [55].

### 3.2.1.3. Poly(ethylene imine) (PEI)

PEI is one of the most potent polymers for gene delivery. PEI is produced by the polymerization of aziridine and has been used to deliver genetic material into various cell types both
"in vitro" and "in vivo" [56,57]. There are two forms of this polymer: the linear form and the
branched form, being the branched structure more efficient in condensing nucleic acids than
the linear PEI [58].

PEI has a high density of protonable amino groups, every third atom being amino nitrogen,
which imparts a high buffering ability at practically any pH [16]. Hence, once inside the endosome, PEI disrupts the vacuole releasing the genetic material in the cytoplasm. This ability to escape from the endosome, as well as the ability to form stable complexes with nucleic
acids, make this polymer very useful as a gene delivery vector [56].

Depending on the type of polymer (e.g. linear or branched PEI), as well as the molecular
weight, the particle sizes of the polyplexes formed are more or less uniformly distributed
[59]. Transfection efficiency of PEI has been found to be dependent on a multitude of factors
such as molecular weight, degree of branching, N/P ratio, complex size, etc [60].

The use of PEI for gene delivery is limited due to the relatively low transfection efficiency,
short duration of gene expression, and elevated toxicity [61,62]. Conjugation of poly(ethylene glycol) to PEI to form diblock or triblock copolymers has been used by some authors to
reduce the toxicity of PEI [63,64,65]. Poly(ethylene glycol) also shields the positive charge of
the polyplexes, thereby providing steric stability to the complex. Such stabilization prevents
non-specific interaction with blood components during systemic delivery [66].

### 3.2.1.4. Dendrimes

Dendrimers are polymer-based molecules with a symmetrical structure in precise size and
shapes, as well as terminal group functionality [8]. Dendrimers contain three regions: i) a
central core (a single atom or a group of atoms having two or more identical chemical fun-
cionalities); ii) branches emanating from core, which are composed of repeating units with
at least one branching junction, whose repetition is organized in a geometric progression
that results in a series of radially concentric layers; and iii) terminal function groups. Dendrimers bind to genetic material when peripheral groups, that are positively-charged at
physiological pH, interact with the negatively-charged phosphate groups of the nucleic acid
[67,68]. Due to their nanometric size, dendrimers can interact effectively and specifically
with cell components such as membranes, organelles, and proteins [69].

For instance, Qi et al. [70] showed the ability of generations 5 and 6 (G5 and G6) of
poly(amidoamine) (PAMAM) dendrimers, conjugated with poly(ethylene glycol) to efficiently transfect both "in vitro" and "in vivo" after intramuscular administration to neonatal
mice. PAMAM has also the ability to deliver siRNAs, especially "in vitro" in cell culture sys-

tems [71-73]. Recent studies showed that the dendrimer-mediated siRNA delivery and gene silencing depends on the stoichiometry, concentration of siRNA and the dendrimer generation [71]. In a recent study, a PAMAM dendrimer-delivered short hairpin RNA (shRNA) showed the ability to deplect a human telomerase reverse transcriptase, the catalytic subunit of telomerase complex, resulting in partial cellular apoptosis, and inhibition of tumor outgrowth in xenotransplanted mice [74].

The toxicity profile of dendrimers is good, although it depends on the number of terminal amino groups and positive charge density. Moreover, toxicity is concentration and generation dependent with higher generations being more toxic as the number of surface groups doubles with increasing generation number [75,76].

### 3.2.1.5. Polymethacrylates

Polymethacrylates are cationic vinyl-based polymers that possess the ability to condense polynucleotides into nanometer size particles. They efficiently condense DNA by forming inter-polyelectrolyte complexes. A range of polymethacrylates, differing in molecular weights and structures, have been evaluated for their potential as gene delivery vector, such us poly[2-dimethylamino) ethyl methacrylate] (DMAEMA) and its co-polymers [16]. The use of polymethactrtylates for DNA transfection is, however, limited due to their low ability to interact with membranes.

In order to optimise the use of these compounds for gene transfer, Christiaens et al. [77] combined polymethacrylates with penetratin, a 16-residue water-soluble peptide that internalises into cells through membrane translocation. Penetratin mainly enhanced the endolysosomal escape of the polymethacrylate–DNA complexes and increased their cellular uptake using COS-1 (kidney cells of the African green monkey). Nanoparticles with a methacrylate core and PEI shell prepared via graft copolymerization have also been employed lately for gene delivery [78,79]. This conjugation resulted in nanoparticles with a higher transfection efficiency and lower toxicity as compared with PEI.

### 3.2.2. Cationic-lipid based non-viral vectors

Cationic lipids have been among the more efficient synthetic gene delivery reagents "in vitro" since the landmark publications in the late 1980s [80]. Cationic lipids can condense nucleic acids into cationic particles when the components are mixed together. This cationic lipid/nucleic acid complex (lipoplex) can protect nucleic acids from enzymatic degradation and deliver the nucleic acids into cells by interacting with the negatively charged cell membrane [81]. Lipoplexes are not an ordered DNA phase surrounded by a lipid bilayer; rather, they are a partially condensed DNA complex with an ordered substructure and an irregular morphology [82,83]. Since the initial studies, hundreds of cationic lipids have been synthesized as candidates for non-viral gene delivery [84] and a few made it to clinical trials [85,86].

Cationic lipids can be used to form lipoplexes by directly mixing the positively charged lipids at the physiological pH with the negatively charged DNA. However, cationic lipids are more frequently used to prepare lipoplex structures such as liposomes, nanoemulsions or solid lipid nanoparticles [81].

### 3.2.2.1. Cationic liposomes

Liposomes are spherical vesicles made of phospholipids used to deliver drugs or genes. They can range in size from 20 nm to a few microns. Cationic liposomes and DNA interact spontaneously to form complexes with 100% loading efficiency; in other words, all of the DNA molecules are complexed with the liposomes, if enough cationic liposomes are available. It is believed that the negative charges of the DNA interact with the positively charged groups of the liposomes [87]. The lipid to DNA ratio, and overall lipid concentration used in forming these complexes, are very important for efficient gene delivery and vary with applications [88].

Liposomes offer several advantages for gene delivery [87]:

- they are relatively cheap to produce and do not cause diseases
- protection of the DNA from degradation, mainly due to nucleases
- they can transport large pieces of DNA
- they can be targeted to specific cells or tissues

Successful delivery of DNA and RNA to a variety of cell types has been reported, including tumour, airway epithelial cells, endothelial cells, hepatocytes, muscle cells and others, by intratissue or intravenous injection into animals [89,90].

Several liposome-based vectors have been assayed in a number of clinical trials for cancer treatment. For instance, Allovectin-7® (Vical, San Diego, CA, USA), a plasmid DNA carrying HLAB and ß2-microglobulin genes complexed with DMRIE/DOPE liposomes have been assessed for safety and efficacy in phase I and II clinical trials [91,92].

### 3.2.2.2. Lipid nanoemulsions

An emulsion is a dispersion of one immiscible liquid in another stabilized by a third component, the emulsifying agent [93]. The nanoemulsion consists of oil, water and surfactants, and presents a droplet size distribution of around 200 nm. Lipid-based carrier systems represent drug vehicles composed of physiological lipids, such as cholesterol, cholesterol esters, phospholipids and tryglicerides, and offer a number of advantages, making them an ideal drug delivery carrier [94]. Adding cationic lipids as surfactants to these dispersed systems makes them suitable for gene delivery. The presence of cationic surfactants, like DOTAP, DOTMA or DC-Chol, causes the formation of positively charged droplets that promote strong electrostatic interactions between emulsion and the anionic nucleic acid phosphate groups [95,96]. For instance, Bruxel et al. [97] prepared a cationic nanoemulsion with DOTAP as a delivery system for oligonucleotides targeting malarial topoisomerase II.

Lipid emulsions are considered to be superior to liposomes mainly in a scaling-up point of view. On the one hand, emulsions can be produced on an industrial scale; on the other hand, emulsions are stable during storage and are highly biocompatible [94]. In addition, the physical characteristics and serum-resistant properties of the DNA/nanoemulsion complexes suggest that cationic nanoemulsions could be a more efficient carrier system for gene and/or immunogene delivery than liposomes. One of the reasons for the serum-resistant properties of the cationic lipid nanoemulsions may be the stability of the nanoemulsion/DNA complex [98]. However, in spite of extensive research on emulsions, very few reports using cationic amino-based nanoemulsions in gene delivery have been published. After "in vivo" administration, cationic nanoemulsions have shown higher transfection and lower toxicity than liposomes [99].

The incorporation of noninonic surfactant with a branched poly(ethylene glycol), such as Tween 80®, increments the stability of the nanoemulsion and prevent the formation of large nanoemulsion/DNA complexes, probably because of their stearic hindrance and the generation of a hydrophilic surface that may enhance the stability by preventing physical aggregation [94]. In addition, this strategy may prevent from enzymatic degradation in blood, and due to the hydrophilic surface, they are taken up slowly by phagocytic cells, resulting in prolonged circulation in blood [100,101].

*3.2.2.3. Solid lipid nanoparticles (SLN)*

Solid lipid nanoparticles are particles made from a lipid being solid at room temperature and also at body temperature. They combine advantages of different colloidal systems. Like emulsions or liposomes, they are physiologically compatible and, like polymeric nanoparticles, it is possible to modulate drug release from the lipid matrix. In addition, SLN possess certain advantages. They can be produced without use of organic solvents, using high pressure homogenization (HPH) method that is already successfully implemented in pharmaceutical industry [102]. From the point of view of application, SLN have very good stability [103] and are subject to be lyophilized [104], which facilitates the industrial production.

Cationic SLN, for instance, SLN containing at least one cationic lipid, have been proposed as non-viral vectors for gene delivery [105,20]. It has been shown that cationic SLN can effectively bind nucleic acids, protect them from DNase I degradation and deliver them into living cells. Cationic lipids are used in the preparation of SLN applied in gene therapy not only due to their positive surface charge, but also due to their surfactant activity, necessary to produce an initial emulsion, which is a common step in most preparation techniques. By means of electrostatic interactions, cationic SLN condense nucleic acids on their surface, leading generally to an excess of positive charges in the final complexes. This is beneficial for transfection because condensation facilitates the mobility of nucleic acids, protects them from environmental enzymes and the cationic character of the vectors allows the interaction with negatively charged cell surface. The characteristics of the resulting complexes depend on the ratio between particle and nucleic acid; there must be an equilibrium between the binding forces of the nucleic acids to SLN to achieve protection without hampering the posterior release in the site of action [106]. Release of DNA from the complexes may be one of the most crucial steps determining the optimal ratio for cationic lipid system-mediated transfection [107].

Our research group showed for the first time the expression of a foreign protein with SLNs in an "in vivo" study [108]. After intravenous administration of SLN containing the EGFP plasmid to BALB/c mice, protein expression was detected in the liver and spleen from the third day after administration, and it was maintained for at least 1 week. In a later study [109], we incorporated dextran and protamine in the SLN and the transfection was improved, being detected also in lung. The improvement in the transfection was related to a longer circulation in the bloodstream due to the presence of dextran on the nanoparticle surface. The surface features of this new vector may also induce a lower opsonization and a slower uptake by the RES. Moreover, the high DNA condensation of protamine that contributes to the nuclease resistance may result in an extended stay of plasmid in the organism. The presence of nuclear localization signals in protamine, which improves the nuclear envelope translocation, and its capacity to facilitate transcription [110] may also explain the improvement of the transfection efficacy "in vivo".

SLN have also been applied for the treatment of ocular diseases by gene therapy. After ocular injection of a SLN based vector to rat eyes, the expression of EGFP was detected in various types of cells depending on the administration route: intravitreal or subretinal. In addition, this vector was also able to transfect corneal cells after topical application [111].

SLN may also be used as delivery systems for siRNA or oligonucleotides. Apolipoprotein-free low-density lipoprotein (LDL) mimicking SLN [112] formed stable complexes with siRNA and exhibited comparable gene silencing efficiency to siRNA complexed with the polymer PEI, and lower citotoxicity. Afterwards, Tao et al. [113] showed that lipid nanoparticles caused 90% reduction of luciferase expression for at least 10 days, after a single systemic administration of 3 mg/kg luciferase siRNA to a liver-luciferase mouse model. CTAB stabilized SLN bearing an antisense oligonucleotide against glucosylceramide synthase (asGCS) reduced the viability of the drug resistant NCI/ADR-RES human ovary cancer cells in the presence of the chemotherapeutic doxorubicin [114].

### 3.2.3. Peptide-based gene non-viral vectors

Many types of peptides, which are generally cationic in nature and able to interact with plasmid DNA through electrostatic interaction, are under intense investigation as a safe alternative for gene therapy [115]. There are mainly four barriers that must be overcome by non-viral vectors to achieve successful gene delivery. The vector must be able to tightly compact and protect DNA, target specific cell-surface receptors, disrupt the endosomal membrane, and deliver the DNA cargo to the nucleus [115]. Peptide-based vectors are advantageous over other non-viral systems because they are able to achieve all of these goals [116]. Cationic peptides rich in basic residues such as lysine and/or arginine are able to efficiently condense DNA into small, compact particles that can be stabilized in serum [117,118]. Attachment of a peptide ligand to a polyplex or lipoplex allows targeting to specific receptors and/or specific cell types. Peptide sequence derived from protein transduction domains are able to selectively lyse the endosomal membrane in its acidic environment leading to cytoplasmic release of the particle [119,120]. Finally, short peptide sequences taken from longer viral proteins can provide nuclear localization signals that help the transport of the nucleic acids to the nucleus [121,122].

### 3.2.3.1. Poly-L-lysine

Poly-L-lysine is a biodegradable peptide synthesized by polimerization on N-carboxy-anhydride of lysine [123]. It is able to form nanometer size complexes with polynucleotides owing to the presence of protonable amine groups on the lysine moiety [16]. The most commonly used poly-L-lysine has a polymerization degree of 90 to 450 [124]. This characteristic makes this peptide suitable for "in vivo" use because it is readily biodegradable [116]. However, as the length of the poly-L-lysine increases, so does the cytotoxicity. Moreover, poly-L-lysine exhibits modest transfection when used alone and requires the addition of an edosomolytic agent such as chloroquine or a fusogenic peptide to allow for release into the cytoplasm. An strategy to prevent plasma protein binding and increase circulation half-life is the attachment of poly(ethylene glycol) to the poly-L-lysine [125,126].

### 3.2.3.2. Peptides in multifunctional delivery systems

Due to the advantages of peptides for gene delivery, they are frequently used to funtionalize cationic lipoplexes or polyplexes. Since these vectors undergo endocytosis, decorating them with endosomolytic peptides for enhanced cytosolic release may be helpful. Moreover, combination with peptides endowed with the ability to target a specific tissue of interest is highly beneficial, since this allows for reduced dose and, therefore, reduced side effects following systemic administration [127]. In a study carried out by our group [19], we improved cell transfection of ARPE-19 cells by using a cell penetration peptide (SAP) with solid lipid nanoparticles. Kwon et al. [128] covalently attached a truncated endosomolytic peptide derived from the carboxy-terminus of the HIV cell entry protein gp41 to a PEI scaffold, obtaining improved gene transfection results compared with unmodified PEI. In other study [20], protamine induced a 6-fold increase in the transfection capacity of SLN in retinal cells due to a shift in the internalization mechanism from caveolae/raft-mediated to clathrin-mediated endocytosis, which promotes the release of the protamine-DNA complexes from the solid lipid nanoparticles; afterwards the transport of the complexes into the nucleus is favoured by the nuclear localization signals of the protamine.

### 3.3. Physical methods for gene delivery

Gene delivery using physical principles has attracted increasing attention. These methods usually employ a physical force to overcome the membrane barrier of the cells and facilitate intracellular gene transfer. The simplicity is one of the characteristics of these methods. The genetic material is introduced into cells without formulating in any particulate or viral system. In a recent publication, Kamimura et al. [87] revised the different physical methods for gene delivery. These methods include the following:

### 3.3.1. Needle injection

The DNA is directly injected through a needle-carrying syringe into tissues. Several tissues have been transfected by this method [87]: muscle, skin, liver, cardiac muscle, and solid tumors. DNA vaccination is the major application of this gene delivery system [129]. The efficiency of needle injection of DNA is low; moreover, transfection is limited to the needle surroundings.

### 3.3.2. Ballistic DNA injection

This method is also called particle bombardment, microprojectile gene transfer or gene gun. DNA-coated gold particles are propelled against cells, forcing intracellular DNA transfer. The accelerating force for DNA-containing particles can be high-voltage electronic discharge, spark discharge or helium pressure discharge. One advantage of this method is that it allows delivering precise DNA doses. However, genes express transiently, and considerable cell damage occurs at the centre of the discharge site. This method has been used in vaccination against the influenza virus [130] and in gene therapy for treatment of ovarian cancer [131].

### 3.3.3. Electroporation

Gene delivery is achieved by generating pores on a cell membrane through electric pulses. The efficiency is determined by the intensity of the pulses, frequency and duration [132]. Electroporation creates transient permeability of the cell membrane and induces a low level of inflammation at the injection site, facilitating DNA uptake by parenchyma cells and antigen-presenting cells [133]. As drawbacks, the number of cells transfected is low, and surgery is required to reach internal organs. This method has been clinically tested for DNA-based vaccination [134] and for cancer treatment [135].

### 3.3.4. Sonoporation

Sonoporation utilizes ultrasound to temporally permeabilize the cell membrane to allow cellular uptake of DNA. It is non-invasive and site-specific and could make it possible to destroy tumor cells after systemic delivery, while leave non-targeted organs unaffected [13]. Gene delivery efficiency seems to be dependent on the intensisty of the pulses, frequency and duration [87]. This method has been applied in the brain, cornea, kidney, peritoneal cavity, muscle, and heart, among others. Low-intensity ultrasonund in combination with microbubbles has recently acquired much attention as a safe method of gene delivery [13]. The use of microbubbles as gene vectors is based on the hypothesis that destruction of DNA-loaded microbubbles by a focused ultrasound beam during their microvascular transit through the target area will result in localized transduction upon disruption of the microbubble shell while sparing non-targeted areas. The therapeutic effect of ultrasound-targeted microbubble destruction is relative to the size, stability, and targeting function of microbubbles.

### 3.3.5. Photoporation

The photoporation method utilizes a single laser pulse as the physical force to generate transient pores on a cell membrane to allow DNA to enter [87]. Efficiency seems to be controlled by the size of the focal point and pulse frequency of the laser. The level of transgene expression reported is similar to that of electroporation. Further studies are needed before this highly sophisticted procedure becomes a practical technique for gene delivery.

### 3.3.6. Magnetofection

This method employs a magnetic field to promote transfection. DNA is complexed with magnetic nanoparticles made of iron oxide and coated with cationic lipids or polymers through electrostatic interaction. The magnetic particles are then concentrated on the target cells by the influence of an external magnetic field. Similar to the mechanism of non-viral vector-based gene delivery, the cellular uptake of DNA is due to endocytosis and pinocytosis [136]. This method has been successfully applied to a wide range of primary cells, and cells that are difficult to transfect by other non-viral vectors [137].

### 3.3.7. Hydroporation

Hydroporation, also called hydrodynamic gene delivery method, is the most commonly method used for gene delivery to hepatocytes in rodents. Intrahepatic gene delivery is achieved by a rapid injection of a large volume of DNA solution via the tail vein in rodents, that results in a transient enlargement of fenestrae, generation of a transient membrane defect on the plasma membrane and gene transfer to hepatocytes [87]. This method has been frequently employed in gene therapy research. In order to apply this simple method of gene administration to the clinic, efforts have been made to reduce the injection volume and avoid tissue damage.

# 4. Strategies to improve transfection mediated by non-viral vectors

The successful delivery of therapeutic genes to the desired target cells and their availability at the intracellular site of action are crucial requirements for efficient gene therapy. The design of safe and efficient non-viral vectors depends mainly on our understanding of the mechanisms involved in the cellular uptake and intracellular disposition of the therapeutic genes as well as their carriers. Moreover, they have to overcome the difficulties after "in vivo" administration.

## 4.1. Target cell uptake and intracellular trafficking

Nucleic acid must be internalized to interact with the intracellular machinery to execute their effect. The positive surface charge of unshielded complexes facilitates cellular internalization. The non-viral vector can be functionalized with compounds that are recognized by the desire specific target cell type. Peptides, proteins, carbohydrates and small molecules have been used to induce target cell-specific internalization [138]. For instance, SLN have been combined with peptides that show penetrating properties, such as the dimeric HIV-1 TAT (Trans-Activator of Transcription) peptide [139] or the synthetic SAP (Sweet Arrow Peptide) [19].

Endocytosis has been postulated as the main entry mechanism for non-viral systems. Various endocytosis mechanisms have been described to date: phagocytosis, pinocytosis, clathrin-mediated endocytosis, caveolae/raft-mediated endocytosis and chathrin and caveolae independent endocytosis. Clathrin-mediated endocytosis leads to an intracellular pathway in which endosomes fuse with lysosomes, which degrade their content, whereas caveolae/raft-mediated endocytosis avoids the lysosomal pathway and its consequent vector degradation [20]. Cytosolic delivery from either endosomes or lisosomes has been reported a major limitation in transfection [140]. In consequence, some research groups have used substances that facilitate endosomal escape before lysosomal degradation. For clathrin-mediated endocytosis, the drop in pH is a useful strategy for endosomal scape via proton destabilization conferred by the cationic carrier, or by pH-dependent activation of membrane disruptive helper molecules, such as DOPE or fusogenic peptides [141-143]. More recently, Leung et al. [144] have patented lipids with 4-amino-butiric acid (FAB) as headgroup to form lipid nanoparticles able to introduce nucleic acids, specifically siRNA, into mammalian cells. FAB lipids also demonstrated membrane destabilizing properties.

Once genes are delivered in the cytoplasm they have to diffuse toward the nuclear region. DNA plasmids have difficulties to diffuse in the cytoplasm because they are large in size. Therefore, packaging and complexing them into small particles facilitates its displacement intracellularly. Diffusion is a function of diameter; hence, smaller particles move faster than larger ones. Thus, another way to optimize gene delivery to the nucleus would be to decrease the size of the particles to increase the velocity of passive diffusion through the cytoplasm [145].

The pass through the nuclear membrane is the next step, and it is in general, quite difficult. There are two mechanisms large molecules can use to overcome that barrier: disruption of the nuclear membrane during mitosis, which is conditioned by the division rate of targeted cells, or import through the nuclear pore complex (NPC). This latter mechanism requires nuclear localization signals, which can be used to improve transfection by non-viral vectors [146]. In this regard, protamine is a peptide that condenses DNA and presents sequences of 6 consecutive arginine residues [147], which make this peptide able to translocate molecules such as DNA from the cytoplasm to the nucleus of living cells. Although protamine/DNA polyplexes are not effective gene vectors [148], the combination of protamine with SLN produced good results in both COS-1 and Na 1330 (murine neuroblastoma) culture cells [149,150]. Precondensation of plasmids with this peptide, to form protamine-DNA complexes that are later bound to cationic SLN, is another alternative that has shown higher transfection capacity in retinal cells compared to SLN prepared without protamine [20].

Once inside the nucleus, level of transgene expression depends on the copy number of DNA and its accessibility for the transcription machinery. Studies have shown that the minimum number of plasmids delivered to the nucleus required for measurable transgene expression depends on the type of vectors [145]. Comparisons between different delivery vehicles showed that higher copy numbers of DNA molecules in the nucleus do not necessarily correlate with higher transfection efficiency. At similar plasmid/nucleus copies, lipofectamine mediated 10-fold higher transfection efficiency than PEI. This suggests that the DNA delivered by PEI is biologically less active than the DNA delivered by lipofectamine. It also emphasizes that a deeper understanding of the nuclear events in gene delivery is required for future progress.

## 4.2. "In vivo" optimization

Vectors mediating high transfection efficiency "in vitro" often fail to achieve similar results "in vivo". One possible reason is that lipidic and polymeric vectors are optimized "in vitro" using two-dimensional (2D) cultures that lack extracellular "in vivo" barriers and do not realistically reflect "in vivo" conditions. While cells "in vitro" grow in monolayers, cells "in vivo" grow in 3D tissue layers held together by the extracellular matrix [145]. This results in cells with reduced thicknesses but larger widths and lengths. Particles that are taken up directly above the nucleus (supranuclear region) have the shortest transport distance to the nucleus and hence a greater chance of delivery success. The spatiotemporal distribution of carriers, however, determines the optimal time for endosomal escape and the optimal intracellular pathway [151]. This highlights the need to develop adequate "in vitro" models that mimics as much as possible the "in vivo" conditions to optimize carriers for gene therapy.

After intravenous administration, plasma nuclease degradation of the nucleic acid is the first barrier that needs to be overcome for therapeutic nucleic acid action. Nucleic acids can be degraded by hydrolytic endo- and exo-nucleases. Both types of nucleases are present in blood. Therefore, increasing nuclease resistance is crucial for achieving therapeutic effects. Naked nucleic acids are not only rapidly degraded upon intravenous injection, they are also cleared from the circulation rapidly, further limiting target tissue localization [138]. To improve nuclease resistance and colloidal stability, complexation strength is an important factor. Shielding the non-viral vectors with poly-L-lysine or poly(ethylene glycol), as mentioned previously, prolongs the circulation time in blood of the vectors.

Vectors delivered "in vivo" by systemic administration not only have to withstand the bloodstream, but also have to overcome the cellular matrix to reach all cell layers of the tissue. While large particles seem to have an advantage "in vitro" due to a sedimentation effect on cells, efficient delivery of particles deep into organs requires particles <100 nm. Small particles (40 nm) diffuse faster and more effectively in the extracellular matrix and inner layers of tissues, whereas larger particles (>100 nm) are restricted by steric hindrance [152].

The net cationic charge of the synthetic vector is a determinant of circulation time, tissue distribution and cellular uptake of synthetic vectors by inducing interactions with negatively blood constituents, such as erythrocytes and proteins. The opsonisation of foreign particles by plasma proteins actually represents one of the steps in the natural process of removal of foreign particles by the innate immune system [153]. This may result in obstruction of small capillaries, possibly leading to serious complication, such as pulmonary embolism [154]. Part of the complexes end up in the reticuoloendothelial system (RES), where they are removed rapidly by phagocytosis or by trapping in fine capillary beds [155]. The nanocarriers, when circulating in blood, can activate the complement system and it seems that the complement activation is higher as the surface charge increases [156,157].

The interaction with blood components is related to the intrinsic properties of the cationic compound (side chain end groups, its spatial conformation and molecular weight), as well as the applied Nitrogen:Phosphate (N:P) ratio [138]. Shielding of the positive surface charge of complexes is currently an important strategy to circumvent the aforementioned problems. The most popular strategy is based on the attachment of water-soluble, neutral, flexible polymers, as poly(ethylene glycol), poly(vinylpyrrolidone) and poly(hydroxyethyl-L-asparagine). The efficacy of the shielding effect of these polymers is determined by the molecular weight and grafting density of the shielding polymer [158]. Longer chains are usually more effective in protecting the particle (surface) from aggregation and opsonisation.

The nanocarriers must arrive to the target tissue to exert their action. Although most commonly used targeting strategies consist of proteins and peptides, carbohydrates have also been utilized [159]. The access of non-viral vector to tumors has been investigated extensively. The discontinuous endothelial cell layer has gaps that give the nanocarriers the opportunity to escape the vascular bed and migrate into the tumoral mass. The most common entities used for tumor targeting include transferrin, epidermal growth factor, and the integrin-binding tripeptide arginine-glycine-aspartic acid (RGD) [159]. Brain targeting has also a great interest; most gene vector do not cross the blood-brain barrier (BBB) after intravenous administration and must be administered through intracerebral injection, which is highly invasive and does not allow for delivery of the gene to other areas of the brain. Injection in the cerebrospinal fluid is also another strategy. Commonly used ligands for mediated uptake are insuline-like growth factors, transferrin or low-density lipid protein [159]. Targeting to the liver has been also investigated in a great extension by many researchers. Carbohydrate-related molecules, such as galactose, asialofetuin, N-acetylgalactosamine and folic acid are the most commonly molecules used for liver targeting [159]. Targeting to endothelial cells provides avenues for improvement of specificity and effectiveness of treatment of many diseases, such as cardiovascular or metabolic diseases [160]. Among other endothelial cell surface determinants, intercellular adhesion molecule-1 (CD54 or ICA-1, a 110-KDa Ig-like transmembrane constitutive endothelial adhesion molecule) is a good candidate target for this goal. ICAM-1 targeting can be achieved by coupling Anti-ICAM-1 antibodies to carriers [161].

## 5. Conclusion

The success of gene therapy is highly dependent on the delivery vector. Viral vectors have dominated the clinical trials in gene therapy for its relatively high delivery efficiency. However, the improvement of efficacy of non-viral vectors has lead to an increased number of products entering into clinical trials. A better understanding of the mechanisms governing the efficiency of transfection, from the formation of the complexes to their intracellular delivery, will lead to the design of better adapted non-viral vectors for gene therapy applications. A number of potentially rate-limiting steps in the processes of non-viral-mediated gene delivery have been identified, which include the efficiency of cell surface association, internalization, release of gene from intracellular compartments such as endosomes, transfer via the cytosol and translocation into the nucleus and transcription efficacy. Insight into molecular features of each of these steps is essential in order to determine their effectiveness as a barrier and to identify means of overcoming these hurdles. Although non-viral vectors may work reasonably well "in vitro", clinical success is still far from ideal. Considering the number of research groups that focus their investigations on the development of new vectors for gene therapy, together with the advances in the development of new technologies to better understand their "in vitro" and "in vivo" behavior, the present limitations of non-viral vectors will be resolved rationally.

## Author details

Alicia Rodríguez Gascón, Ana del Pozo-Rodríguez and María Ángeles Solinís

*Address all correspondence to: alicia.rodriguez@ehu.es

Pharmacokinetics, Nanotechnology and Gene Therapy Group, Faculty of Phamacy, University of the Basque Country UPV/EHU, Spain

## References

[1] Venter JC, Adams MD, Myers EW, et al. The Sequence of the Human Genome. Science 2001;291(5507) 1304-51.

[2] Kassner PD. Discovery of Novel Targets with High Throughput RNA Interference Screening. Combinatorial Chemistry & High Throughput Screen 2008;11(3) 175-184.

[3] Wiltgen M, Tilz GP. DNA Microarray Analysis: Principles and Clinical Impact. Hematology 2007;12(4) 27-87.

[4] Directive 2009/120/EC of the European Parliament. http://eur-lex.europa.eu/LexUriServ/LexUriServ.do?uri=OJ:L:2009:242:0003:0012:EN:PDF (accessed 07 August 2012).

[5] Zhang Y, Satterlee A, Huang L. In Vivo Gene Delivery by Nonviral Vectors: Overcoming Hurdles?. Molecular Therapy 2012; 20(7) 1298-1304.

[6] Gene Therapy Clinical Trials Worldwide.Provided by the Journal of Gene Medicine. Jon Wiley and Sons Ltd, 2012; http://www.wiley.co.k/genmed/clinical (accessed 01 August 2012).

[7] Li SD, Huang L. Non-viral is Superior to Viral Gene Delivery. Journal of Controlled Release 2007;123(3) 181-183.

[8]  Pérez-Martinez FC, Carrión B, Ceña V. The Use of Nanoparticles for Gene Therapy in the Nervous System. Journal of Alzheimer's Disease 2012;31(4) 697-710.

[9]  Roy I, Mitra S, Maitra A, Mozumdar S. Calcium Phosphate Nanoparticles as Novel Non-viral Vectors for Targeted Gene Delivery. International Journal of Pharmaceutics 2003;250(1) 25-33.

[10]  Armatas GS, Kanatzidis MG. Mesostructured Germanium with Cubic Pore Symmetry. Nature 2006;441(7097) 1122-1125.

[11]  Zou X, Conradsson T, Klingstedt M, Dadachov MS, O'Keeffe M. A Mesoporous Germanium Oxide with Crystalline Pore Walls and its Chiral Derivative. Nature 2005;437(7059) 716-719.

[12]  Slowing II, Vivero-Escoto JL, Wu CW, Lin VS. Mesoporous Silica Nanoparticles as Controlled Release Drug Delivery and Gene Transfection Carriers. Advanced Drug Delivery Reviews 2008;60(11) 1278-1288.

[13]  Guo X, Huang L. Recent Advances in Nonviral Vectors for Gene Delivery. Accounts of Chemical Research 2012;45(7) 971-979.

[14]  Skolova V, Epple M. Inorganic Nanoparticles as Carriers of Nucleic Acids into Cells. Angewandte Chemie International Edition 2008;47(8) 1382-1395.

[15]  Bhattarai SR, Muthuswamy E, Wani A, et al. Enhanced Gene and siRNA Delivery by Polycation-Modified Mesoporous Silica Nanoparticles Loaded with Chloroquine. Pharmaceutical Research 2010;27(12) 2556-2568.

[16]  Basarkar A, SinghJ. Nanoparticulate Systems for Polynucleotide Delivery. International Journal of Nanomedicine 2007;2(3) 353-360.

[17]  Yamashita S, Fukushima H, Akiyama Y, et al. Controlled-Release System of Single Stranded DNA Triggered by the Photothermal Effect of Gold Nanorods and its In Vivo Application. Bioorganic & Medicinal Chemistry 2011;19(7) 2130-2135.

[18]  Raviña M, Cubillo E, Olmeda D, et al. Hyaluronic Acid/Chitosan-g-poly(ethylene glycol) Nanoparticles for Gene Therapy: an Application for pDNA and siRNA Delivery. Pharmaceutical Research 2010;27(12) 2544-2555.

[19]  del Pozo-Rodríguez A, Pujals S, Delgado D, et al. A Proline-Rich Peptide Improves Cell Transfection of Solid Lipid Nanoparticle-Based Non-Viral Vectors. Journal of Controlled Release 2009;133(1) 52-59.

[20]  Delgado D, del Pozo-Rodríguez A, Solinís MA, Rodríguez-Gascón A. Understanding the Mechanism of Protamine in Solid Lipid Nanoparticle-Based Lipofection: the Importance of the Entry Pathway. European Journal of Pharmaceutics and Biopharmaceutics 2011;79(3) 495-502.

[21]  Nie H, Khew ST, Lee LY, Poh KL, Tong YW, Wang C-H. Lysine-Based Peptide-Functionalized PLGA Foams for Controlled DNA Delivery. Journal of Controlled Release 2009;138(1) 64-70.

[22] Luten J, van Nostrum CF, De Smedt SC, Hennink WE. Biodegradable Polymers as Non-Viral Carriers for Plasmid DNA Delivery. Journal of Controlled Release 2008;126(2) 97-110.

[23] Bala I, Hariharan S, Kumar M. PLGA Nanoparticles in Drug Delivery: The State of the Art. Critical Reviews in Therapeutics Drug Carrier Systems 2004;21(5) 387–422.

[24] Panyam J, Labhasetwar V. Biodegradable Nanoparticles for Drug and Gene Delivery to Cells and Tissue. Advanced Drug Delivery Reviews 2003;55(3) 329–347.

[25] Shive MS, Anderson JM. Biodegradation and Biocompatibility of PLA and PLGA Microspheres. Advanced Drug Delivery Reviews 1997;28(1) 5–24.

[26] Wang D, Robinson DR, Kwon GS, Samuel J. Encapsulation of Plasmid DNA in Biodegradable poly(D,L-lactic-co-glycolic acid) Microspheres as a Novel Approach for Immunogene Delivery. Journal of Controlled Release 1999;57(1) 9–18.

[27] Banchereau J, Steinman RM. Dendritic Cells and the Control of Immunity. Nature 1998;392(6673) 245–252.

[28] Walter E, Dreher D, Kok M, et al. Hydrophilic poly(DL lactide- co-glycolide) Microspheres for the Delivery of DNA to Human-Derived Macrophages and Dendritic cells. Journal of Controlled Release 2001;76(1-2)149–168.

[29] Singh M, Ugozzoli M, Briones M, Kazzaz J, Soenawan E, O'Hagan DT. The Effect of CTAB Concentration in Cationic PLG Microparticles on DNA Adsorption and In Vivo Performance. Pharmaceutical Research 2003;20(2) 247–251.

[30] Walker E, Moelling K, Pavlovic J, Merkle HP. Microencapsulation of DNA Using poly(DL-lactide-co-glycolide): Stability Issues and Release Characteristics. Journal of Controlled Release 1999;61(3) 361-374.

[31] Kusonowiriyawong C, Atuah K, Alpar OH, Merkle HP, Walter E. Cationic Stearylamine-Containing Biodegradable Microparticles for DNA Delivery. Journal of Microencapsulation 2004;21(1) 25-36.

[32] Benoit MA, Ribet C, Distexhe J, et al. Studies on the Potential of Microparticles Entrapping pDNA-poly(aminoacids) Complexes as Vaccine Delivery Systems. Journal of Drug Targeting 2001;9(4) 253-266.

[33] Nie Y, Zhang ZA, Duan YR. Combined Use of Polycationic Peptide and Biodegradable Macromolecular Polymer as a Novel Gene Delivery System: a Preliminary Study. Drug Delivery 2006;13(6) 441-446.

[34] Pérea C, Sánchez A, Putnam D, Ting D, Langer R, Alonso MJ. Poly(lactic acid)-poly(ethylene glycol) Nanoparticles as New Carriers for the Delivery of Plasmid DNA. Journal of Controlled Release 2001;75(1) 211-224.

[35] Shinde RR, Bachmann MH, Wang Q, Kasper R, Contag CH. PEG-PLA/PLGA Nanoparticles for In-Vivo RNAi Delivery. Nanotech: conference technical proceedings, May 20-23, 2007, Santa Clara Convention Centar, Santa Clara, California, USA.

[36] Hong L, Wei N, Joshi V, et al. Effects of Glucocorticoid Receptor Small Interfering RNA Delivered Using Poly Lactic-co-Glycolic Acid Microparticles on Proliferation and Differentiation Capabilities of Human Mesenchymal Stromal Cells. Tissue Engineering Part A 2012;18 (7-8) 775-784.

[37] Zheng F, Shi XW, Yang GF, et al. Chitosan Nanoparticle as Gene Therapy Vector Via Gastrointestinal Mucosa Administration: Results of an In Vitro and In Vivo Study. Life Sciences 2007;80(4) 388–396.

[38] Hejazi R, Amiji M. Chitosan-based Gastrointestinal Delivery Systems. Journal of Controlled Release 2003;89(2) 151–165.

[39] Rao SB, Sharma CP. Use of Chitosan as a Biomaterial: Studies on its Safety and Hemostatic Potential. Journal of Biomedical Materials Research 1997;34(1) 21–28.

[40] Aspden TJ, Mason JD, Jones NS, Lowe J, Skaugrud O, Illum L. Chitosan as a Nasal Delivery System: the Effect of Chitosan Solution on In Vitro and In Vivo Mucociliary Transport Rates in Human Turbinates and Volunteers. Journal of Pharmaceutical Sciences 1997;86(4) 509–513.

[41] Fang N, Chan V, Mao HQ, Leong KW. Interactions of Phospholipid Bilayer with Chitosan: Effect of Molecular Weight and pH. Biomacromolecules 2001;2(4) 1161–1168.

[42] Cui Z, Mumper RJ. Chitosan-based Nanoparticles for Topical Genetic Immunization. Journal of Controlled Release 2001;75(3) 409–419.

[43] Takeuchi H, Yamamoto H, Niwa T, Hino T, Kawashima Y. Enteral Absorption of Insulin in Rats from Mucoadhesive Chitosan-coated Liposomes. Pharmaceutical Research 1996;13(6) 896–901.

[44] Illum L. Chitosan and its Use as a Pharmaceutical Excipient. Pharmaceutical Research 1998;15(9) 1326–1331.

[45] Leong KW, Mao HQ, Truong-Le VL, Roy K, Walsh SM, August JT. DNA-Polycation Nanospheres as Non-Viral Gene Delivery Vehicles. Journal of Controlled Release 1998;53(1) 183–193.

[46] Csaba N, Köping-Höggård M, Fernandez-Megia E, Novoa-Carballal R, Riguera R, Alonso MJ. Ionically Crosslinked Chitosan Nanoparticles as Gene Delivery Systems: Effect of PEGylation Degree on In Vitro and In Vivo Gene Transfer. Journal of Biomedical Nanotechnology 2009;5(2) 162–171.

[47] de la Fuente M, Seijo B, Alonso MJ. Bioadhesive Hyaluronan-Chitosan Nanoparticles can Transport Genes Across the Ocular Mucosa and Transfect Ocular Tissue. Gene Therapy 2008;15(9) 668–676.

[48] de la Fuente M, Seijo B, Alonso MJ. Novel Hyaluronic Acid-Chitosan Nanoparticles for Ocular Gene Therapy. Investigative Ophthalmology & Visual Science 2008;49(5) 2016–2024.

[49]  Katas H, Alpar HO. Development and Characterisation of Chitosan Nanoparticles for siRNA Delivery. Journal of Controlled Release 2006;115(2) 216–225.

[50]  Garcia-Fuentes M, Alonso MJ. Chitosan-based Drug Nanocarriers: Where do we Stand?.Journal of Controlled Release 2012;161(2) 496-504

[51]  Rojanarata T, Opanasopit P, Techaarpornkul S, Ngawhirunpat T, Ruktanonchai U. Chitosan-Thiamine Pyrophosphate as a Novel Carrier for siRNA Delivery. Pharmaceutical Research 2008;25(12) 2807–2814.

[52]  Ji AM, Su D, Che O, et al. Functional Gene Silencing Mediated by Chitosan/siRNA Nanocomplexes. Nanotechnology 2009;20(40) 405103.

[53]  Yuan Q, Shah J, Hein S, Misra RD. Controlled and Extended Drug Release Behaviour of Chitosan-based Nanoparticle Carrier. Acta Biomaterialia 2010;6(3) 1140–1148.

[54]  Huang M, Fong CW, Khor E, Lim LY. Transfection Efficiency of Chitosan Vectors: Effect of Polymer Molecular Weight and Degree of Deacetylation. Journal of Controlled Release 2005;106(3) 391–406.

[55]  Kiang T, Wen J, Lim HW, Leong KW. The Effect of the Degree of Chitosan Deacetylation on the Efficiency of Gene Transfection. Biomaterials 2004;25(22) 5293–5301.

[56]  Boussif O, Lezoualc'h F, Zanta MA et al. A Versatile Vector for Gene and Oligonucleotide Transfer into Cells in Culture and In Vivo: Polyethylenimine. Proceedings of the National Academy of Sciences of the United States of America 1995;92(16) 7297-7301.

[57]  Abdallah B, Hassan A, Benoist C, Goula D, Behr JP, Demeneix BA. A Powerful Non-viral Vector for In Vivo Gene Transfer into the Adult Mammalian Brain: Polyethylenimine. Human Gene Therapy 1996;7(16) 1947-1954.

[58]  Dunlap DD, Maggi A, Soria MR, Monaco L. Nanoscopic Structure of DNA Condensed for Gene Delivery. Nucleic Acids Research 1997;25(15) 3095-3101.

[59]  Debus H, Beck-Broichsitter M, Kissel T. Optimized Preparation of pDNA/poly(ethyleneimine) Polyplexes Uusing a Microfluidic System. Lab on a Chip 2012;12(14) 2498-2506.

[60]  Thomas M, Ge Q, Lu JJ, et al. Cross-Linked Small Polyethylenimines: While Still Nontoxic, Deliver DNA Efficiently to Mammalian Cells In Vitro and In Vivo. Pharmaceutical Research 2005;22(3) 373-380.

[61]  Chollet P, Favrot MC, Hurbin A, Coll JL. Side-Effects of a Systemic Injection of Linear Polyethylenimine-DNA Complexes. The Journal of Gene Medicine 2002;4(1): 84-91.

[62]  Moghimi SM, Symonds P, Murray JC, Hunter AC, Debska G, Szewczyk A. A Two-stage Poly(ethylenimine)-Mediated Cytotoxicity: Implications for Gene Transfer/ Therapy. Molecular Therapy 2005;11(6) 990-995.

[63]  Choi HS, Ooya T, Yui N. One-Pot Synthesis of a Polyrotaxane Via Selective Thread-
      ing of a PEI-b-PEG-b-PEI Copolymer. Macromolecular Biosciences 2006;6(6) 420-424.

[64]  Park MR, Han KO, Han IK, et al. Degradable Polyethyleneimine-alt-poly(ethylene
      glycol) Copolymers as Novel Gene Carriers. Journal of Controlled Release
      2005;105(3) 367-380.

[65]  Zhong Z, Feijen J, Lok MC, et al. Low Molecular Weight Linear Polyethyleneimine-
      bpoly(ethylene glycol)-b-polyethylenimine Triblock Copolymers: Synthesis, Charac-
      terization, and In Vitro Gene Transfer Properties. Biomacromolecules 2005;6(6)
      33440-33448.

[66]  Kursa M, Walker GF, Roessler V et al. Novel Shielded Transferring-Polyethylene
      Glycol-Polyethylenimine/DNA Complexes for Systemic Tumor-Targeted Gene
      Transfer. Bioconjugate Chemistry 2003;14(1) 222-231.

[67]  Nandy B, Santosh M, Maiti PK. Interaction of Nucleic Acids with Carbon Nanotubes
      and Dendrimers Journal of Biosciences 2012;37(3) 457–474.

[68]  Lee H, Larson RG. Lipid Bilayer Curvature and Pore Formation Induced by Charged
      Linear Polymers and Dendrimers: the Effect of Molecular Shape. The Journal of
      Physical Chemistry B 2008;112(39) 12279–12285.

[69]  Dutta T, Jain NK, McMillan NA, Parekh HS. Dendrimer Nanocarriers as Versatile
      Vectors in Gene Delivery. Nanomedicine 2010;6(1) 25–34.

[70]  Qi R, Gao Y, Tang Y et al. PEG-conjugated PAMAM Dendrimers Mediate Efficient
      Intramuscular Gene Expression. The AAPS Journal 2009;11(3): 395–405.

[71]  Liu X, Huang H, Wang J et al. Dendrimers-Delivered Short Hairpin RNA Targeting
      hTERT Inhibits Oral Cancer Cell Growth In Vitro and In Vivo. Biochemical Pharma-
      cology 2011;82(1) 17-23.

[72]  Khurana B, Goyal AK, Budhiraja A, Arora D, Vyas SP. siRNA Delivery Using Nano-
      carriers - an Efficient Tool for Gene Silencing. Current Gene Therapy 2010;10(2)
      139-155.

[73]  Pavan GM, Albertazzi L, Danani A. Ability to Adapt: Different Generations of PA-
      MAM Dendrimers show Different Behaviors in Binding siRNA. The Journal of Physi-
      cal Chemistry B 2010;114 (8) 2667–2675.

[74]  Liu X, Huang H, Wang J et al. Dendrimers-Delivered Short Hairpin RNA Targeting
      hTERT Inhibits Oral Cancer Cell Growth In Vitro and In Vivo. Biochemical Pharma-
      cology 2011;82(1) 17-23.

[75]  Choi YJ, Kang SJ, Kim YJ, Lim YB, Chung HW. Comparative Studies on the Genotox-
      icity and Cytotoxicity of Polymeric Gene Carriers Polyethylenimine (PEI) and Polya-
      midoamine (PAMAM) Dendrimer in Jurkat T-cells. Drug and Chemical Toxicology
      2010;33(4) 357–366.

[76] Duncan R, Izzo L. Dendrimer Biocompatibility and Toxicity. Advanced Drug Delivery Reviews 2005;57 (15) 2215–2237

[77] Christiaens B, Dubruel P, Grooten J, et al. Enhancement of Polymethacrylate-Mediated Gene Delivery by Penetratin. European Journal of Pharmaceutical Sciences 2005;24(5) 525-537.

[78] Li P, Zhu JM, Sunintaboom P, Harris FW. New Route to Amphiphilic Core-Shell Polymer Nanospheres: Graft Copolymerization of Methyl Methacrylate from Water-Soluble Polymer Chains Containing Amino Groups. Langmuir 2002;18(22) 8641-8646.

[79] Feng M, Lee D, Li P. Intracellular Uptake and Release of Poly(ethyleneimine)-copoly(methyl methacrylate) Nanoparticle/pDNA Complexes for Gene Delivery. International Journal of Pharmaceutics 2006;311(1-2) 209-214.

[80] Felgner PL, Gadek TR, Holm M, et al. Lipofection: a Highly Efficient, Lipid-Mediated DNA-Transfection Procedure. Proceedings of the National Academy of Sciences of the United States of America 1987;84(21) 7413-7417.

[81] Gascon AR, Pedraz JL. Cationic Lipids as Gene Transfer Agents: a Patent Review. Expert Opinion on Therapeutic Patents 2008;18(5) 515-524.

[82] Xu Y, Hui SW, Frederik P, Szoka FC Jr. Physicochemical Characterization and Purification of Cationic Lipoplexes. Biophysical Journal 1999;77(1) 341-353.

[83] Radler JO, Koltover I, Salditt T, Safinya CR. Structure of DNA-Cationic Liposome Complexes: DNA Intercalation in Multilamellar Membranes in Distinct Interhelical Packing Regimes. Science 1997;275(5301) 810-814.

[84] Mahato RI., ed. Kim SW. Pharmaceutical Perspectives of Nucleic Acid-Based Therapeutics. London: Taylor & Francis; 2002.

[85] Edelstein ML, Abedi MR, Wixon J, Edelstein RM. Gene Therapy Clinical Trials Worldwide 1989-2004 - an Overview. The Journal of Gene Medicine 2004;6(6) 597-602.

[86] Edelstein ML, Abedi MR, Wixon J. Gene Therapy Clinical Trials Worldwide to 2007 – an Update. The Journal of Gene Medicine 2007;9(10) 833-842.

[87] Kamimura K, Suda T, Zhang G, Liu D. Advances in gene delivery systems. Pharmaceutical Medicine 2011;25(5) 293-306.

[88] Zhou X, Huang L. DNA Transfection Mediated by Cationic Liposomes Containing Lipopolylysine: Characterization and Mechanism of Action. Biochimica et Biophysica Acta 1994;1189(2) 195-203.

[89] Xu L, Huang CC, Huang W, et al. Systemic Tumor-Targeted Gene Delivery by Antitransferrin Receptor scFv-Immunoliposomes. Molecular Cancer Therapeutics 2002;1(5) 337-346.

[90] Pardridge WM. Re-engineering Biopharmaceuticals for Delivery to Brain with Molecular Trojan Horses.Bioconjugate Chemistry 2008;19(7) 1327-1338.

[91] Stopeck AT, Hersh EM, Akporiaye ET, et al. Phase I Study of Direct Gene Transfer of an Allogeneic Histocompatibility Antigen, HLA-B7, in Patients with Metastatic Melanoma. Journal of Clinical Oncology 1997;15(1) 341-349.

[92] Stopeck AT, Jones A, Hersh EM, et al. Phase II Study of Direct Intralesional Gene Transfer of Allovectin-7, an HLA-B7/beta2-microglobulin DNA-Liposome Complex, in Patients with Metastatic Melanoma. Clinical Cancer Research 2001;7(8): 2285–2291.

[93] Becher P., ed. Emulsions, Theory and Practice. New York: Reinhold; 1965.

[94] Verissimo LM, Lima LF, Egito LC, de Oliveira AG, do Egito ES. Pharmaceutical Emulsions: a New Approach for Gene Therapy. Journal of Drug Targeting 2010;18(5) 333-342.

[95] Martini E, Fattal E, de Oliveira MC, Teixeira H. Effect of Cationic Lipid Composition on Properties of Oligonucleotide/emulsion Complexes: Physico-chemical and Release Studies. International Journal of Pharmaceutics 2008;352(1–2) 280–286.

[96] Marty R, N'soukpoé-Kossi CN, Charbonneau D, Weinert CM, Kreplak L, Tajmir-Riahi HA. Structural Analysis of DNA Complexation with Cationic Lipids. Nucleic Acids Research 2009;37(3) 849–857.

[97] Bruxel F, Cojean S, Bochot A, et al. Cationic Nanoemulsion as a Delivery System for Oligonucleotides Targeting Malarial Topoisomerase II. International Journal of Pharmaceutics 2011;416(2) 402-409.

[98] Yi SW, Yune TY, Kim TW, et al. A Cationic Lipid Emulsion/DNA Complex as a Physically Stable and Serum-Resistant Gene Delivery System. Pharmaceutical Research 2000;17(3) 314-320.

[99] Kwon SM, Nam HY, Nam T, et al. In Vivo Time-Dependent Gene Expression of Cationic Lipid-Based Emulsion as a Stable and Biocompatible Non-Viral Gene Carrier. Journal of Controlled Release 2008;128(1) 89-97.

[100] Buyens K, Demeester J, De Smedt SS, Sanders NN. Elucidating the Encapsulation of Short Interfering RNA in PEGylated Cationic Liposomes. Langmuir 2009;25(9) 4886-4891.

[101] Kim TW, Kim YJ, Chung H, Kwon IC, Sung HC, Jeong SY. The Role of Non-Ionic Surfactants on Cationic Lipid Mediated Gene Transfer. Journal of Controlled Release 2002;82(2-3) 455-465.

[102] Teeranachaideekul V, Müller RH, Junyaprasert VB. Encapsulation of Ascorbylpalmitate in Nanostructured Lipid Xarriers (NLC)--Effects of Formulation Parameters on Physicochemical Stability. International Journal of Pharmaceutics 2007;340(1-2) 198-206.

[103]  Müller R, Mäder K, Gohla S. Solid Lipid Nanoparticles (SLN) for Controlled Drug Delivery - a Review of the State of the Art. European Journal of Pharmaceutics and Biopharmaceutics 2000; 50(1) 161-177.

[104]  del Pozo-Rodríguez A, Solinís MA, Gascón AR, Pedraz JL. Short- and Long-Term Stability Study of Lyophilized Solid Lipid Nanoparticles for Gene Therapy. EuropeanJournal of Pharmaceutics and Biopharmaceutics 2009;71(2) 181-189.

[105]  del Pozo-Rodríguez A, Delgado D, Solinís MA, Gascón AR, Pedraz JL. Solid Lipid Nanoparticles: Formulation Factors Affecting Cell Transfection Capacity. International Journal of Pharmaceutics 2007;339(1-2) 261-268.

[106]  del Pozo-Rodríguez A, Delgado D, Solinís MA, Gascón AR. Lipid Nanoparticles as Vehicles for Macromolecules: Nucleic Acids and Peptides. Recent Patents on Drug Delivery & Formulation 2011;5(3) 214-226.

[107]  Sakurai F, Inoue R, Nishino Y, Okuda A, Matsumoto O, Taga T. Effect of NA/Liposome Mixing Ratio on the Physicochemical Characteristics, Cellular Uptake and Intracellular Trafficking of Plasmid DNA/Cationic Liposome Complexes and Subsequent Gene Expression. Journal of Controlled Release 2000;66(2-3) 255-269.

[108]  del Pozo-Rodríguez A, Delgado D, Solinís MA, et al. Solid Lipid Nanoparticles as Potential Tools for Gene Therapy: In Vivo Protein Expression After Intravenous Administration. International Journal of Pharmaceutics 2010;385(1-2) 157-162.

[109]  Delgado D, Gascón AR, del Pozo-Rodríguez A, et al. Dextran-Protamine-Solid Lipid Nanoparticles as a Non-Viral Vector for Gene Therapy: In Vitro Characterization and In Vivo Transfection after Intravenous Administration to Mice. International Journal of Pharmaceutics 2012;425(1-2) 35-43.

[110]  Masuda T, Akita H, Harashima H. Evaluation of Nuclear Transfer and Transcription of Plasmid DNA Condensed with Protamine by Microinjection: the Use of a Nuclear Transfer Score. FEBS Letters 2005;579(10) 2143-2148.

[111]  Delgado D, del Pozo-Rodríguez A, Solinís MA, et al. Dextran and Protamine-based Solid Lipid Nanoparticles as Potential Vectors for the Treatment of X-linked Juvenile Retinoschisis. Human Gene Therapy 2012;23(4) 345-355.

[112]  Kim HR, Kim IK, Bae KH, Lee SH, Lee Y, Park TG. Cationic Solid Lipid Nanoparticles Reconstituted from Low Density Lipoprotein Components for Delivery of siRNA. Molecular Pharmaceutics 2008;5(4) 622-631.

[113]  Tao W, Davide JP, Cai M, et al. Noninvasive Imaging of Lipid Nanoparticle-Mediated Systemic Delivery of Small-Interfering RNA to the Liver. Molecular Therapy 2010;18(9) 1657-1666.

[114]  Siddiqui A, Patwardhan GA, Liu YY, Nazzal S. Mixed Backbone Antisense Glucosylceramide Synthase Oligonucleotide (MBO-asGCS) Loaded Solid Lipid Nanoparticles: In Vitro Characterization and Reversal of Multidrug Resistance in NCI/ADR-RES Cells. International Journal of Pharmaceutics 2010;400(1-2) 251-259.

[115]  Mahato RI. Nonviral Peptide-based Approaches to Gene Delivery. Journal of Drug Targeting 1999;7(4) 249-268.

[116]  Martin ME, Rice KG. Peptide-guided Gene Delivery. The AAPS Journal 2007;9(1) E18-E29.

[117]  Adami RC, Rice KG. Metabolic Stability of Glutaraldehyde Cross-linked Peptide DNA Condensates. Journal of Pharmaceutical Sciences 1999;88(8) 739-746.

[118]  McKenzie DL, Kwok KY, Rice KG. A Potent New Class of Reductively Activated Peptide Gene Delivery Agents. The Journal of Biological Chemistry 2000;275(14) 9970-9977.

[119]  Gupta B, Levchenko TS, Torchilin VP. Intracellular Delivery of Large Molecules and Small Particles by Cell-Penetrating Proteins and Peptides. Advanced Drug Delivery Reviews 2005; 57(4) 637-651.

[120]  Deshayes S, Morris MC, Divita G, Heitz F. Cell-Penetrating Peptides: Tools for Intracellular Delivery of Therapeutics. Cellular and Molecular Life Science 2005;62(16) 1839-1849.

[121]  Goldfarb DS, Gariepy J, Schoolnik G, Kornberg RD. Synthetic Peptides as Nuclear Localization signals. Nature.1986;322(6080) 641-644.

[122]  Nigg EA. Nucleocytoplasmic Transport: Signals, Mechanisms and Regulation. Nature. 1997;386(6627) 779-787.

[123]  Zhang S, Xu Y, Wang B, Qiao W, Liu D, Li Z. Cationic Compounds Used in Lipoplexes and Polyplexes for Gene Delivery. Journal of Controlled Release 2004;100(2) 165-180.

[124]  Wadhwa MS, Collard WT, Adami RC, McKenzie DL, Rice KG. Peptide-Mediated Gene Delivery: Influence of Peptide Structure on Gene Expression. Bioconjugate Chemistry 1997;8(1) 81-88.

[125]  El-Aneed A. An Overview of Current Delivery Systems in Cancer Gene Ttherapy. Journal of Controlled Release 2004;94(1) 1-14.

[126]  Tiera MJ, Winnik FO, Fernandes JC. Synthetic and Natural Polycations for Gene Therapy: State of the Art and New Perspectives. Current Gene Therapy 2006;6(1) 59-71.

[127]  Hoyer J, Neundorf I. Peptide Vectors for the Nonviral Delivery of Nucleic Acids. Accounts of Chemical Research 2012;45(7) 1048-1056.

[128]  Kwon EJ, Liong S, Pun SH. A Truncated HGP Peptide Sequence that Retains Endosomolytic Activity and Improves Gene Delivery Efficiencies. Molecular Pharmaceutics 2010;7(4) 1260-1265.

[129]  Prausnitz MR, Mikszta JA, Cormier M, Andrianov AK. Microneedle-based Vaccines. Current Topics in Microbiology and Immunology 2009;333 369-393.

[130] Yager EJ, Dean HJ, Fuller DH. Prospects for Developing an Effective Particle-Mediated DNA Vaccine Against influenza. Expert Review of Vaccines. 2009;8(9) 1205-1220.

[131] Kaur T, Slavcev RA, Wettig SD. Addressing the Challenge: Current and Future Directions in Ovarian Cancer Therapy. Current Gene Therapy 2009;9(6) 434-458.

[132] Heller LC, Ugen K, Heller R. Electroporation for Targeted Gene Transfer. Expert Opinion on Drug Delivery 2005;2(2) 255-268.

[133] van DrunenLittel-van den Hurk S, Hannaman D. Electroporation for DNA Immunization: Clinical Application. Expert Review of Vaccines 2010;9(5) 503-517.

[134] Bodles-Brakhop AM, Heller R, Draghia-Akli R. Electroporation for the Delivery of DNA-based Vaccines and Immunotherapeutics: Current Clinical Developments. Molecular Therapy 2009;17(4) 585-592.

[135] Heller R, Jaroszeski MJ, Glass LF, et al. Phase I/II Trial for the Treatment of Cutaneous and Subcutaneous Tumors using Electrochemotherapy. Cancer 1996;77(5) 964-971.

[136] Plank C, Anton M, Rudolph C, Rosenecker J, Krötz F. Enhancing and Targeting Nucleic Acid Delivery by Magnetic Force. Expert Opinion on Biological Therapy 2003;3(5) 745-758.

[137] Mykhaylyk O, Antequera YS, Vlaskou D, Plank C. Generation of Magnetic Nonviral Gene Transfer Agents and Magnetofection In Vitro. Nature Protocols 2007;2(10) 391-2411.

[138] Schiffelers RM, de Wolf HK, van Rooy I, Storm G. Synthetic Delivery Systems for Intravenous Administration of Nucleic Acids. Nanomedicine 2007;2(2)169-181.

[139] Rudolph C, Schillinger U, Ortiz A, et al. Application of Novel Solid Lipid Nanoparticle (SLN)-Gene Vector Formulations Based on a Dimeric HIV-1 TAT-Peptide In Vitro and In Vivo. Pharmaceutical Research 2004;21(9) 1662-1669.

[140] El-Sayed A, Futaki S, Harashima H. Delivery of Macromolecules Using Arginine-Rich Cell-Penetrating Peptides: Ways to Overcomes Endosomal Entrapment. The AAPS Journal 2009;11(1) 13-22.

[141] Choi SH, Jin SE, Lee MK, et al. Novel Cationic Solid Lipid Nanoparticles Enhanced p53 Gene Transfer to Lung Cancer Cells. European Journal of Pharmaceutics and Biopharmaceutics 2008;68(3) 545-554.

[142] Dincer S, Turk M, Piskin E. Intelligent Polymers as Nonviral Vectors. Gene Therapy 2005;12(1) S139-S145.

[143] Yessine MA, Leroux JC. Membrane-Destabilizing Polyanions: Interaction with Lipid Bilayers and Endosomal Escape of Biomacromolecules. Advanced Drug Delivery Reviews 2004;56(7) 999-1021.

[144] Leung KK, Masuna S, Ciufolini M, Cullis PR. Reverse Head Group Lipids, Lipid Compositions Comprising Reverse Headgroup Lipids, and Methods for Delivery of Nucleic Acids. WO2011056682; 2011.

[145] Nguyen J, Szoka FC. Nucleic Acid Delivery: the Missing Pieces of the Puzzle? Accounts of Chemical Research 2012;45(7) 1153-1162.

[146] Boulanger C, Di Giorgio C, Vierling P. Synthesis of Acridine-Nuclear Localization Signal (NLS) Conjugates and Evaluation of their Impact on Lipoplex and Polyplex-based Ttransfection. European Journal of Medicinal Chemistry 2005;40(12) 1295-1306.

[147] Biegeleisen K.The Probable Structure of the Protamine-DNA Complex. Journal of Theoretical Biology 2006;241(3) 533-540.

[148] Xu Z, Gu W, Chen L, Gao Y, Zhang Z, Li Y. A Smart Nanoassembly Consisting of Acid-Labile Vinyl Ether PEG-DOPE and Protamine for Gene Delivery: Preparation and "In Vitro" Transfection. Biomacromolecules 2008;9(11) 3119-3126.

[149] Vighi E, Ruozi B, Montanari M, Battini R, Leo E. pDNA Condensation Capacity and In Vitro Gene Delivery Properties of Cationic Solid Lipid Nanoparticles. International Journal of Pharmaceutics 2010;389(1-2) 254-261.

[150] Vighi E, Montanari M, Ruozi B, Tosi G, Magli A, Leo E. Nuclear Localization of Cationic Solid Lipid Nnanoparticles Containing Protamine as Transfection Promoter. European Journal of Pharmaceutics and Biopharmaceutics 2010;76(3) 384-393.

[151] Dinh AT, Pangarkar C, Theofanous T, Mitragotri S. Understanding Intracellular Transport Processes Pertinent to Synthetic Gene Delivery Via Stochastic Simulations and Sensitivity Analyses. Biophysical Journal 2007;92(3) 831-846.

[152] Ng CP, Pun SH. A Perfusable 3D Cell-Matrix Tissue Culture Chamber for In Situ Evaluation of Nanoparticle Vehicle Penetration and Transport. Biotechnology and Bioengineering 2008;99(6) 1490-1501.

[153] Owens DE 3rd, Peppas NA. Opsonization, Biodistribution, and Pharmacokinetics of Polymeric Nanopartices. International Journal of Pharmaceutics 2006;307(1) 93-102.

[154] Ogris M, Brunner S, Schuller S, Kircheis R, Wagner E. PEGylated DNA Transferring-PEI Complexes: Reduced Interaction with Blood Components, Extended Circulation in Blood and Potential for Systemic Gene Delivery. Gene Therapy 1999;6(4) 595-605.

[155] Merdan T, Kopeced J, Kissel T. Prospects for Cationic Polymers in Gene and Oligonucleotide Therapy Against Cancer. Advanced Drug Delivery Reviews 2002;54(5) 715-758.

[156] Moghimi SM, Szebeni J. Stealth Liposomes and Long Circulating Nanoparticles: Critical Issues in Pharmacokinetics, Opsonisation and Protein-Binding Properties. Progress in Lipid Research 2003;42(6) 463-478.

[157] Krieg AM. CpG Motifs in Bacterial DNA and their Iimmune Effects. Annual Review of Immunology 2002;20 709-760.

[158] Kunath K, von Harpe A, Petersen H, et al. The Structure of PEG-Modified Poly(ethyl-eneimines) Influences Biodistribution and Pharmacokinetics of their Complexes with NF-kappaB Decoy in mice. Pharmaceutical Research 2002;19(6) 810-817.

[159] Viola JR, El-Andaloussi S, Oprea II, Smith CI. Non-viral Nanovectors for Gene Delivery: Factors that Govern Successful Therapeutics. Expert Opinion on Drug Delivery 2010;7(6) 721-735.

[160] Muro S, Dziubla T, Qiu W, et al. Endothelial Targeting of High-Affinity Multivalent Polymer Nanocarriers Directed to Intercellular Adhesion Molecule 1. The Journal of Pharmacology and Experimental Therapeutics 2006;317(3) 1161-1169.

[161] Koren E, Torchilin VP. Drug Carriers for Vascular Drug Delivery. IUBMB Life 2011;63(8) 586-595.

# Chapter 2

# Silencing of Transgene Expression: A Gene Therapy Perspective

Oleg E. Tolmachov, Tatiana Subkhankulova and Tanya Tolmachova

Additional information is available at the end of the chapter

## 1. Introduction

The treatment of a number of diseases can be achieved through gene addition therapy, where curative transgenes are established within the patient's cells after delivery with viral or non-viral vectors. The defective cells requiring treatment are typically differentiated; these cells or their progenitors can be targeted for therapeutic gene transfer. However, as the abundance of progenitor cells varies between different tissues and in the same tissue during the fetal, neonatal and adult stages of development, the scarcity of a particular progenitor cell pool, the paucity of spontaneous departures of progenitor cells down differentiation pathways and unclear differentiation induction conditions can complicate genetic therapeutic intervention via these cells. Nevertheless, gene transfer to progenitor cells can be a preferred option when differentiated cells are either poorly accessible for the vector or, once differentiated, are defective beyond repair by gene therapy. Genetic conditions with considerable value in therapeutic gene transfer to progenitor cells include cystic fibrosis (CF) and severe combined immunodeficiency (SCID).

The delivered transgenes can integrate into the chromosomal DNA, replicate episomally or persist as non-replicating episomal elements in non-dividing cells. Depending on the properties of the transgene expression cassette, particular features of specific transgene integration sites and the state of the individual recipient cells, the transgenes are expressed with varying degree of efficiency. On some occasions, the transgenes are permanently silenced immediately after introduction, on other occasions transgene silencing occurs only after a certain period of adequate expression and on still other occasions transgene expression varies dramatically among the individual clones of transgene-harbouring cells. Such variation is thought to be mainly due to the transgene's interaction with its immediate genetic neighbourhood within the host genome; a phenomenon, which is similar to 'position effect variegation' in normal development caused by spontaneous clone-wise silencing of some resident genes [1]. Typical position effect variegation is epigenetic instability and should be distinguished from variegation due to somatic mutations, e.g. due to variations in the length of polynucleotide repeat expansions [2] or due to the sorting of mitochondrial genomes in mitochondrial heteroplasmia [3]. The element of randomness, which is inherently present in position effect variegation, should not come as a surprise. In fact, stochastic fluctuations of gene expression are typical both at the level of variation between different cells of tissue and at the level of temporal variation within one cell. Both of these modes of variation are essential for normal differentiation and tissue-patterning with the input of stochastic variation being decisive when a developmental signal is present at a near-critical level. For the gene therapist, it is important that the permanent silencing of transgene expression can occur both in postmitotic target cells and target cells undergoing clonal expansion, while variegation is typically associated with clones of dividing cells. Stable long-term transgene expression in differentiating cells is particularly challenging. In fact, the introduced genes are subject to the pre-existing and developing gene expression patterns in the target cells, which can override the signals from the transgenes' own regulatory elements and, thus, can cause transgene expression shutdown. Indeed, at a transcriptional level, the changing scenery of transcription initiation factor pools, chromatin re-modelling and DNA methylation events during differentiation contribute to the transiency of transgene expression.

Genomes in general and, in particular, mammalian genomes have a mosaic organisation with functionally related genetic elements often being in close physical proximity. There are three teleological reasons for this: 1) expediency of genetic exchange; 2) straightforward temporal control of gene expression; 3) economy of energy, enzymes and other factors serving the genetic elements. The second and the third of these reasons are also sufficient for the existence of a finely patterned 3D-arrangement of DNA in interphase nuclei, simplifying the functional interactions between distant genetic elements, e.g. interactions regulating gene expression. It is intriguing to propose that the need to orchestrate gene expression in time and the economy need are also driving the astonishing interconnectedness of all gene silencing mechanisms, which we shall address in this chapter.

The gene therapist should take advantage of the pre-existing regulatory moduli present in the target cells and should also supply the transgenes with their own expression control elements. The regulatory elements required for reliable, long-term and tissue-specific transgene expression include minimal promoters, enhancers, regulatory introns and locus control regions. The functional arrangement of all these elements is ultimately achieved in 3D. This should be borne in mind, when 2D assemblies of regulatory elements are called 'promoters'. Some 'promoters' are, in fact, motley artificial chimeras. For example, a fusion between a human cytomegalovirus (CMV) immediate-early enhancer and chicken beta-actin promoter, exon1 and intron1 is called 'CBA promoter' or 'CAG promoter' [4].

In general, in the majority of situations in gene therapy, transgene silencing and variegation are undesirable. We review here different factors, both host-dependent and vector-dependent, which are known to contribute to silencing and variegation of transgene expression and which should be taken into account where choosing or designing effective gene therapy vectors and strategies for their administration.

# 2. Host genetic factors of silencing and position effect variegation

Patterns for maintaining gene repression or activation are governed by regulatory machinery acting at multiple levels: 1) transcription; 2) mRNA processing, export from the nucleus, translation and degradation; 3) protein folding, modification, transport and degradation. Control of gene expression is well-coordinated and highly hierarchical, with the control of transcription initiation situated at the top of the regulatory ladder. A number of interacting instruments of transcriptional gene activation and silencing in mammals are known: DNA methylation (e.g. methylation within CpG-islands of promoters), amino acid sequence variants of histones, covalent modifications of histones, histone-binding proteins (e.g. powerful inhibitors of gene activity from the Polycomb Group) and combinations of transcription initiation factors specific for particular tissues and developmental stages. The pivotal point is the access of the transcription machinery to DNA, which is regulated via DNA methylation and chromatin remodelling. With some simplification, it can be generalized that 'coarse tuning' of gene expression (e.g. long-term silencing) is provided by DNA methylation, 'medium tuning' is provided by chromatin remodelling and 'fine tuning' is achieved via various transcription factors and a multitude of other regulatory devices.

The various branches of the regulatory machinery play their own particular roles and yet are inherently interconnected. As detailed below, a prime example of this is the deep involvement of the miRNA pathway both in mRNA degradation and in the establishment of chromatin methylation patterns [5].

## 2.1. The role of DNA methylation in silencing

DNA methylation is an important epigenetic mark involved in cell differentiation and organ and tissue development, which plays a crucial role in the establishment of genomic imprinting (parent-dependent silencing of alternative alleles) in both male and female germ lines. However, in gene transfer experiments, the methylation of transgenes was shown to be just one ingredient in the dynamic interplay of various factors responsible for silencing and variegation [6].

*De-novo* methylation patterns in humans are established mainly on implantation and in gametogenesis. Two DNA (cytosine-5)-methyltransferases, DNMT3A and DNMT3B, play an essential role in *de-novo* methylation while DNMT3A in cooperation with the auxiliary protein DNMT3L is responsible for imprinting. There is still much we do not know about the manner in which the inactive state of the imprinted chromosomal domains is achieved and what factors trigger this type of silencing. The available evidence indicates that 'Smc hinge proteins' can be particularly important in epigenetic silencing [7]. Thus, in studies based on X-linked GFP transgene silencing, the SmcHD1 gene was shown to play a critical role in X-chromosome inactivation in mammals [8,9]. The recruitment of SmcHD1 to the X-chromosome may involve the non-coding Xist RNA, proteins from the Polycomb group and DNA methyltransferases [7].

An area of intriguing research is the relationship between DNA hypermethylation and the function of locus control regions (LCRs), controlling the local state of chromatin [10,11].

## 2.2. The role of histone variants and histone modifications in silencing

There are two types of structural variations among histone molecules. Firstly, there are low abundance species of histones with unusual amino acid sequences, so-called histone variants. Secondly, histones are amenable to standard covalent protein modifications such as acetylations and methylations of specific amino acid residues. Both structural variations are known to play important roles in the regulation of gene expression activity.

Regions of constitutive heterochromatin are particularly prone to encroaching on the transgene in a variable pattern in different cells and, thus, to interfering with transgene expression. Different loci in human chromosomes have a variable tendency to become involved in heterochromatin structures. For example, chromosomes' centromeres and telomeres are typical regions of heterochromatin, which are known to expand occasionally, inducing steady or intermittent silencing. In the case of centromeres, the silencing machinery might involve the histone variant CENP-A, which is found exclusively in centromeres. Other histone variants could also play a role in silencing. Thus, the histone variant macroH2A appears to be important in gene silencing on the inactive X-chromosome. In contrast, the histone variants H2A.Z and H3.3 are known to be conducive for transcription.

DNA methylation and histone modifications are closely linked to chromatin remodelling and are often jointly implicated in gene silencing and position effect variegation. Using an *in vivo* mammalian model for position effect variegation, Hiragami-Hamada and co-workers [12] extensively investigated the molecular basis for the stability of heterochromatin-mediated silencing in mammals. Comparison between two transgenic lines, containing different numbers of copies of human CD2 transgenes integrated within or close to a block of the pericentric heterochromatin, revealed that the variegation of CD2 expression is indeed associated with both genomic DNA methylation and histone modifications such as H3K9me3. However, DNA methylation was the key modification that accompanied the formation of an inaccessible chromatin structure and more stable gene silencing [12,13].

## 2.3. Silencing mediated by Polycomb proteins

Silencing can be mediated by proteins from the Polycomb group (PcG). These proteins can form giant complexes, which are tethered to histones and regulatory DNA sequences called Polycomb Response Elements (PREs). When the PcG proteins bind histones, they suppress all the gene expression activity in the respective area of chromatin. In mammals, PcG proteins are known to be involved in cell differentiation and tissue formation and also to contribute to tumorigenesis, genomic imprinting, stem cell maintenance and aging [14-16]. The emerging picture from fundamental research suggests that counteracting PcG repression can only be achieved by a combination of multiple inputs converging at chromatin [17]. Besides the normal requirement for the recruitment of transcription factors and co-activators, the genomic targets of PcG proteins require the activity of specific demethylases and methyltransferases for the gene expression to proceed [18].

Importantly for gene therapy, PcG protein complexes have been recently demonstrated to be able to repress transcription activity in genomic repeats and some transgenes [19].

### 2.4. Tissue specific and developmental stage specific transcription factors

There are two types of transcription factors: 1) auxiliary proteins, which bind other proteins in the transcription complex; 2) DNA-binding sequence-specific transcription factors. The latter type can straightforwardly be recognised *in silico* by the observation of some distinct patterns within the DNA-binding domains of transcription factors, e.g. the zinc-finger motif, the helix-loop-helix motif or the leucine-zipper motif. *In silico* analysis, e.g. using *Biobase* software (http://www.biobase-international.com), is currently also a method of choice for pinpointing transcription factor binding sites and, therefore, for predicting gene expression activation patterns.

### 2.5. Silencing mediated by non-coding RNAs

It has become clear that non-coding RNAs have an important bearing on gene and transgene expression. In general, there are several mechanisms for the regulatory effects of non-coding RNAs in gene expression. The two most important control points appear to be the direct regulation of transcription initiation and the regulation of mRNA degradation through RNAi by miRNAs. Recent findings revealed that non-coding RNAs are critical factors in the recruitment of PcG members to the cell chromatin [20,21]. At the same time, the miRNA pathway turned out to be significant in establishing the DNA methylation and histone modification patterns [5,22].

In animals, small RNAs, namely piRNA species, which are typically 24-32 nucleotides in length, have been shown to mediate genomic DNA methylation. These non-coding RNAs associate with Piwi clade proteins from the Argonaut superfamily and act analogously to the well-documented RdMD complexes in plants. The primary role of piRNA in many animals appears to be the silencing of retrotransposones via DNA methylation in germ lines. In fact, the lack of transposons' suppression in spermatogenesis often results in defects and the loss of germ cells with age. Although it is not clear whether the same mechanism is responsible for the protective silencing of viral genomes after viral infections of mammalian cells, the small RNAs are likely to be involved in *de-novo* methylation of viral DNA through a similar mechanism. Thus, small noncoding RNAs could potentially provide a flexible regulatory link between transgene recognition, PcG proteins recruitment and transgene silencing through DNA methylation, histone modifications and chromatin remodelling.

It appears that, in general, regulation via RNAi has a smaller long-term influence on gene expression than histone modifications and DNA methylation, acting rather as a rapid response system. Indeed, it would be too energetically inconvenient for cells to synthesize mRNA and then to destroy it on a permanent basis.

## 3. Gene vector properties, which are known to contribute to transgene silencing

Long-term transgene expression is highly desirable for most gene therapy applications. However, it is a relatively common occurrence for transgene expression to die out both in terms of the decrease of the efficiency of expression in individual cells and in terms of the reduction of the fraction of expressing cells.

A wide variety of vectors can be used for the delivery and establishment of transgenes and their control elements. Some of the vectors, so called 'viral vectors', are generated using a top-down approach by piggy-backing on the natural gene transfer machinery of viruses. In contrast, 'non-viral' vectors are either pure nucleic acids or synthetic nano-particles, which are generated using a bottom-up strategy. A pivotal feature of any gene therapy vector (with the obvious exception of cytoplasmic-only vectors such as mRNA-based vectors) is the final localization of the delivered transgenes in the nuclei of the target cells. In general, transgenes can be integrated into random chromosomal sites, integrated into pre-selected chromosomal sites and/or left to exist episomally. Specialized molecular machinery for efficient random integration is born by retroviral vectors [23], lentiviral vectors and eukaryotic transposon vectors. Although the bulk of the DNA delivered with non-transposable plasmid, minicircle and PCR-generated vectors stays episomally, some of the vector DNA also randomly integrates into the chromosomal DNA. The genetic neighbourhood at a transgene integration site has an important bearing on the temporal profile of transgene expression. Nevertheless, many factors that determine the susceptibility of transgene to silencing are defined by the properties of the employed vector, transgene and co-introduced expression control elements.

Multimeric transgene inserts were reported to induce silencing [24]. Unfavourably, even if a gene vector delivers monomeric DNA, spontaneous chromosomal integrations often result in vector DNA multimers (it remains unclear whether the multimers are formed before or after the initial integration event). Silencing due to repetitive DNA was also demonstrated when the introduced DNA contained trinucleotide repeat expansions [25]. This result has an implication for the gene therapy of recessive polyglutamine diseases, as therapeutic transgenes can contain triplet expansions of some minimal length. The precise mechanism for silencing through the recognition of multimeric transgenes and trinucleotide repeats in the host genomic DNA still remains unclear.

Transgene silencing is often blamed on the malfunction of foreign gene expression control elements. Indeed, this phenomenon is sometimes referred to as 'promoter shut down'. Certainly, different promoters vary in their ability to maintain long-term transgene expression in specific cell populations. In particular, there is a clear tendency for some promoters to turn off in cells where they are not normally active. The mechanisms for such effects can be quite indirect. Thus, the ubiquitous CMV promoter can activate transgene expression in antigen-presenting cells with the ensuing immune response and elimination of all vulnerable transgene expressing cells [26].

Some bacterial plasmid backbones are known to cause transgene silencing [27-29]. In addition, bacterial plasmid backbones interfere with gene delivery into human cells after DNA administration *in vivo* because of the innate TLR9-receptor-mediated immune reaction to unmethylated bacterial 'CpG-motifs' within these backbones. In an attempt to alleviate the immune reaction, methylation of these sequences *in vitro* was attempted. Disappointingly, on some occasions the methylation of plasmid gene vector DNA resulted in increased silencing of transgene expression [30]. The depletion or ablation of CpG motifs from bacterial plasmid backbones is known to substantially reduce their immunogenicity. The effects of CpG-depletion and ablation on transgene silencing are expected, but the available data on this issue are currently quite limited.

Bacterial lypopolysaccharides (LPS) often co-purify and contaminate plasmid gene vector DNA. These endotoxins can substantially reduce the efficiency of transfection *in vitro* [31,32] and *in vivo*, where LPS are known to induce a TLR4-receptor-mediated innate immune response. Bacterial endotoxins exhibit a profound effect on cellular regulatory networks [33]. Therefore, it is possible that tilting cells towards 'transgene-silencing mode' is an important contributing factor in the endotoxin-mediated inhibition of transfection.

## 4. Therapeutic gene vectors and the strategies for their use, which are employed to avoid transgene silencing

Stable long-term transgene expression depends on the intertwined issues of reliable maintenance of transgenes in target cells and a robust policy to prevent undesired transgene silencing. In general, these two issues are to a large extent under the control of the gene therapist, as both of them can be addressed through the gene vector design and the delivery mode. The regulation of gene expression in eukaryotic cells is exceptionally complex and multi-faceted. As a result, the strategies used to achieve sustainable transgene expression should address multiple possible reasons for the transgene expression shutdown.

### 4.1. Employment of cytoplasmic-only (non-nuclear) vectors

As most silencing mechanisms are nuclear-based, gene vectors with direct cytoplasmic expression, which are not required to enter the nucleoplasm, are well-positioned to avoid silencing. Thus, non-viral mRNA vectors [34] or positive strand RNA-based viral vectors such as Sendai virus based vectors [35] can be employed. In addition to the escape from silencing, the advantages of extra-nuclear-delivery vectors include relatively fast transgene expression and the absence of potentially mutagenic genomic insertions. The downside is that transgene expression using such vectors is never long-term because of the eventual degradation of RNA in cells and because of RNA dilution in the dividing cells. Moreover, the fundamentally low fidelity of RNA replication undermines efforts to generate artificial vector systems with replicating RNA episomes. The key upside is that low immunogenicity and minimal toxicity of such vectors accommodate their repeated administration well.

## 4.2. CpG ablation, CpG depletion and minimized DNA vectors

The methylation of chromosomal DNA is one of the most powerful mechanisms for the shut-down of gene expression. Thus, the design of gene therapy vectors should take into account the amenity of the vector sequences to methylation. Firstly, the purposeful exclusion of entire methylation-prone CpG islands should be considered. Secondly, CpG-depleted or CpG-ablated modules, produced through the point-wise replacement or removal of CpG dinucleotides, should be taken advantage of. The generation of functionally active CpG-ablated sequences is fairly laborious; the CpG-ablated gamma replicon from the bacterial plasmid R6K and some antibiotic-resistance genes are available from *Invivogen*.

Clearly, as repetitive sequences are known to induce silencing, their use in therapeutic gene vectors should be avoided as far as possible.

A common way to reduce the chances of transgene silencing is to shorten the auxiliary vector sequences outside of the therapeutic transgene expression cassette. For example, the plasmid selection markers can be very short indeed [36]. In fact, a plasmid replication origin can be re-utilised as a plasmid marker using the 'plasmid addiction' phenomenon [37].

The trend to exclude unwanted sequences from gene transfer vectors led to the generation of specialized minimized DNA vectors. The most tested versions of such vectors are DNA fragments amplified *in vitro* using polymerase chain reaction (PCR) [38], plasmid-derived linear terminally looped 'midges'   [39] or circular supercoiled 'minicircles' [40]. Minicircle vectors are produced by intramolecular site-specific recombination within bacterial plasmids. The superior efficiency of gene delivery and the longevity of transgene expression achieved with minicircle DNA was observed in multiple studies (e.g. [41]). The production of minimized DNA vectors is a biotechnological challenge. For example, advanced methods and bacterial strains were developed for efficient bacteria-based minicircle DNA production. The generation of PCR amplicons with Taq-polymerase is relatively inexpensive. However, the load of Taq-polymerase-introduced mutations may make one consider alternative *in vitro* amplification methods for the large-scale synthesis of double-stranded DNA, e.g. ligase chain reaction (LCR), which is based on the ligation of preassembled oligonucleotides.

The usual aim in the production of minimized DNA vectors is the removal of sequences of bacterial origin, such as plasmid backbone sequences, as they can be immunogenic and some of them were reported to cause silencing [27,29]. It should be emphasized that transgene silencing through the co-delivery of specific plasmid sequences should not be generalized to all plasmid sequences and each plasmid sequence or bacterial sequence needs to be tested individually. More research is required to identify the affected bacterial replicons and to pinpoint the mechanism for the induction of silencing by bacterial DNA sequences. Another avenue is the development of novel specialized forms of minimized vectors, such as 'minivectors' for RNAi-based therapy [42].

### 4.3. Judicious choice of tissue-specific, inducible and ubiquitous promoters to control transgene expression

Promoters are the gene expression control elements, which are typically co-introduced with therapeutic transgenes. In scientific literature, the word 'promoter' is often an umbrella term, which in addition to a minimal promoter also incorporates other linked genetic elements such as enhancers, transcription factor binding sites and even regulatory introns. Promoter is a key element of the regulatory machinery required for long-term non-silenced transgene expression. Different promoters vary in their strength, tissue specificity, specificity for particular developmental stages and ability to react to external stimuli (inducibility). Each therapeutic setting requires a thoughtful choice of a transgene promoter. Thus, some ubiquitous promoters are appropriate for consistent long-term transgene expression in differentiating stem cells passing through a number of developmental phases [43]. Ubiquitous promoters are also appropriate in situations where the resident homologue of the therapeutic gene is naturally expressed ubiquitously [44]. Tissue-specific promoters have been known for a long time to be instrumental for long-term transgene expression in terminally differentiated cells in the liver, vascular tissue, muscle and central nervous system [45]. Inducible promoters are appropriate where the constitutive expression of the therapeutic transgene is undesired and/or where bespoke activation of the therapeutic transgene is required. In addition to the heavily used tetracycline-sensing promoter systems, inducible promoters can be activated by heat, light and gas-born acetaldehyde [46]. Clearly, the construction and determined exploitation of new hybrid promoters can resolve many issues in transgene silencing.

### 4.4. Multiple transgene insertions into random chromosomal sites

Random integration of transgenes into chromosomes is typical for a number of gene delivery systems. Spontaneous chromosomal integration of vector DNA within target cells is not efficient. Thus, enhanced random chromosomal integration of plasmid gene vectors can be attained using genetic elements of eukaryotic transposons, retroviruses or lentiviruses (lentiviruses form a subgroup of retroviruses with a somewhat larger genome and the ability to infect non-dividing cells). However, many integration events occur in unfavourable genetic neighbourhoods resulting in the silencing of the respective copies of the transgenes. Hence, position-dependent silencing means that individual transfected or transduced cell clones differ in terms of the longevity of the transgene expression. Random chromosomal integration of transgenes tend to occur in transcriptionally active areas of the genome where heterochromatin condensation and DNA methylation are unlikely to interfere with transgene expression. However, as cells differentiate, the pattern of heterochromatization and DNA methylation changes and some of the transgenes find themselves in transcriptionally silent areas of the genome. Therefore, the shutdown of transgene expression is particularly common in cell populations undergoing differentiation. In these circumstances, it is certainly possible to increase the chances of long-term transgene expression by increasing the number of randomly chromosomally integrated transgenes through a higher concentration of vector and/or repeated rounds of vector administration. Thus, the gene therapist can aim to generate multiple copies of transgenes, indiscriminately integrated within the target genome, hoping that at least one of the copies will reside in a suitable chromosomal site that will be immune to silencing.

The employment of transposable genetic elements for efficient random integration of therapeutic transgenes was complicated by the fact that mammals do not have their own active or easily re-activatable transposons. Therefore, a number of heterologous transposons were adapted for use in human cells. Recombination machinery from Sleeping Beauty, PiggyBac, Tol2 and Mos1 transposons was shown to be capable of directing chromosomal integration of transgenes [47]. Genes for transposases were either included within the cargo gene vector plasmid or were delivered into human cells on a separate plasmid. Mutant transposases with enhanced activity for random DNA integration were developed.

A caveat of the anti-silencing strategy relying on multiple transgene insertions into random chromosome sites is a possibility of potentially deleterious or tumourigenic mutations due to insertional mutagenesis. However, this drawback is irrelevant for highly differentiated and non-dividing cells where, firstly, only a limited set of gene products is required for cell survival and functional competence and, secondly, only a minimal risk is present for the selection of malignancies. In fact, many terminally differentiated cells are either polyploid or polynucleated; both of these statuses can alleviate the impact of insertional mutagenesis.

### 4.5. Site-specific chromosomal integration

One of the ideal scenarios, where transgene silencing is avoided, involves the transgene DNA being site-specifically integrated into a 'benign', silencing-resistant chromosomal site where there is little chance of transgene consumption by heterochromatin. Thus, targeting transgenes to a continuously active chromosomal locus can resolve the transgene expression shutdown problem. In particular, sites could exist within chromosomal DNA, where an integrated transgene would be immune to chromatin re-arrangements and other regulatory events during differentiation. A possible candidate site is the human homologue of mouse Rosa 26 locus, which is being successfully used to express various transgenes in mouse transgenic studies.

In principle, both transposases and retroviral integrases can be re-engineered into site-directed recombination enzymes through their fusion with appropriate site-specific 'tethering' domains [48]. In addition to tethered transposases and retroviral integrases, the site-specific integration of transgenes into human chromosomes can be achieved via the modification of *bona fide* site-specific recombination systems.

Site-specific DNA recombination systems are comprised of recombinase enzymes, their cofactors and their cognate recombination sites. Site-specific recombination systems can be classified into two general types: irreversible and reversible ones.

Site-specific recombination machinery for irreversible recombination is typically borrowed from the chromosome integration systems of temperate bacteriophages. In integrative recombination systems there are two types of recombination sites, which are normally referred to as *attP* and *attB*. An archetypical example is bacteriophage lambda integrase (Int)

catalysing a one-off recombination event between the lambda's *attP* site and the chromosomal *attB* site. The reverse reaction, excision of prophage, is often possible; however, a separate enzyme or a separate subunit of bacteriophage integrase is normally required to
catalyze the excision. The *attB* sites are typically shorter than the corresponding *attP* sites.
Thus, in the recombination system from the *Streptomyces coelicolor* bacteriophage phiC31,
*attP* is 39 bp long and *attB* is 34 bp long. Similarly, the recombination system from the *Lacto-
coccus lactis* bacteriophage TP901-1 has 50 bp long *attP* and 31 bp long *attB*. Consequently, in
artificial recombination systems within the mammalian setting, higher specificity of integration is achieved with longer *attP* sites positioned within the chromosomal loci. It has turned
out that the human genome contains a close analogue of the phiC31 *attP* site. Extensive mutagenesis of the phiC31 integrase gene has produced versions of the enzymes with very high
specific activity towards this native human site [49]. Cell-permeable and nuclear targeted
versions of phiC31 integrase were also created, these recombinant enzymes can be used to
create transient, 'hit-and-run', recombinase activity in human cells that is required for the
stable integration of therapeutic transgenes.

The typical original *in vivo* function of the reversible site-specific recombination systems is
to preserve the monomeric status of a plasmid, prophage or episome via the resolution of
circular DNA multimers to monomers; monomeric status is important for the maintenance
stability of many plasmid replicons. Commonly used reversible systems include bacteriophage's P1Cre recombinase with its cognate *loxP* sites and FLP recombinase (flipase) with its
cognate *FTR* sites from the yeast *Saccharomyces cerevisiae* '2-micron circle' episome. Many reversible systems were successfully used for the chromosomal integration of transgenes in
pre-engineered cells. However, it should be noted that some site-specific recombination systems are fundamentally unsuitable for chromosomal integration strategies. Thus, ParA re-
solvase and *MRS* sites from the plasmid RK2 constitute a reversible system for
intramolecular recombination; however, in this system there is no molecular recombination
between *MRS* sites situated on separate DNA molecules.

Of course, the employed bacterial recombination systems have to be functional in eukaryotic
cells [50]. A potential pitfall to be aware of is that some of the site-specific recombinases require an additional co-factor; e.g., IHF (integration host factor) is an obligatory element for
lambda Int/*attB*/*attP* system. Unexpectedly and encouragingly, at least on some occasions
mammalian cells are able to provide suitable co-factors [50].

The wild type human adeno-associated virus type 2 (AAV2) is the only known human virus
capable of site-specific chromosomal integration. AAV2 uses the chromosome-tethering
strategy for genomic insertions. Expression of the Rep gene is required for integration of the
viral genome into a unique DNA sequence within specific chromosomal loci. The Rep proteins of this virus bind both several Rep Binding Sites (RBS) within the viral DNA and the
RBS sites in the human genome (known as AAVS1, AAVS2 and AAVS3) leading to preferential integration of the viral DNA in the genomic loci 19q13.42, 5p13.3 and 3p24.3.

An important step forward in the exploitation of the site-specific integration system of AAV
was achieved when the AAV Rep protein was used to direct the integration of integrase-defective retroviral vectors into human 19q13.42 locus [51]. The transfer of the locus-specific

chromosomal integration apparatus of AAV2 to other vector types, e.g., plasmid gene vectors, can be accomplished as well [52].

### 4.6. Episomal localisation of a transgene

Episomal maintenance of transgene expression cassettes is an attractive strategy to escape the control of some resident gene regulation systems, such as chromatin remodelling machinery, over transgene expression. The problem with this approach is that viral replicons, e.g., compact episomal replicons from SV40, polyoma, papilloma viruses, which are often completely adequate for the research use of gene vectors, are rarely acceptable for therapeutic applications. Indeed, the expression of the large SV40 T-antigen and, hence, the malignant transformation of the recipient host cells is required for SV40-origin-based replication. Similarly, EBNA1-oriP DNA segment of Epstein-Barr Virus (EBV) can be used to support the maintenance of plasmid gene vectors in the nucleoplasm of dividing laboratory cells. Although EBNA1 expression does not result in a typical malignant transformation, it can still tilt the cells towards undesired immortalisation [53].

Alternative benign episomal replicons are being sought. Encouragingly, the scaffold/ matrix attachment region (S/MAR) from the human β-interferon gene was reported to support non-viral episomal replication when coupled to a promoter [54]. Thus, episomal maintenance mediated by S/MAR elements might be the reason behind the well-established beneficial effects of these elements on transgene expression [41,55,56]. Non-viral episomal vectors also include mammalian artificial chromosomes (MACs), which can be generated through both top-down and bottom-up approaches [57,58]. However, current progress with MACs is limited because of prohibiting costs associated with the generation of these vectors.

### 4.7. Employment of the locus control regions within the vectors

Protection of integrated transgenes from encroaching heterochromatin can be achieved with chromatin insulators or other *cis*-acting locus control regions (LCRs) [59]. The mechanistic details of LCRs action are currently not clear and so the terminology in this area is somewhat diffuse with, for example, 'chromatin boundary elements' and 'chromatin insulators' often being used synonymously [60,61]. Some enhancers have an important bearing on the state of chromatin and, therefore, can also be viewed as LCRs. Experiments with some known chromatin insulators show that their effects on transgene expression are not always positive and to a large extent depend on the cell context [62,63]. Nuclear 'matrix attachment region' elements (MARs) and the effectively synonymous nuclear 'scaffold attachment region' elements (SARs) are known to possess some LCR activity. Some authors are trying to avoid the confusion between MARs and SARs using the joined names 'SAR/MARs', 'MAR/ SARs' or 'S/MARs'. Promising results in terms of sustained transgene expression were achieved with MARs both within the scenario where two MAR elements are used 'to protect the transgene from the flanks' [64,65] and the scenario where a single promoter-MAR couple is driving the transgene's episomal replication [41].

## 4.8. Top-up transgene administration to compensate for silenced transgenes

Normally, if the expression of therapeutic transgenes did die out, it is possible to perform a new round of gene transfer, thus achieving a new burst of transgene expression. Repeated vector administration can be particularly sought-after when the target cell population experiences programmed death, while the respective progenitor cell pool is poorly accessible for therapeutic gene transfer. This strategy can be used without hesitation in an *ex vivo* gene therapy setting where therapeutic genes are delivered *in vitro* to dividing cells derived from a patient's biopsy prior to autologous transplantation. In contrast, in an *in vivo* gene therapy setting, the drawbacks of vector re-administration include not only the increased complexity and cost of treatment, but also the realistic possibilities that immunity to elements of the vector might develop and that the effects of the toxic elements of the vector might build up to an unacceptable level. That is why low immunogenicity, low toxicity and the biodegradability of auxiliary vector elements are important in the vector re-administration treatment format.

## 4.9. Selection of clones with stable non-silenced transgene expression

Reliable, robust and error-free site-specific integration into mammalian cells lacking pre-engineered integration sites is difficult to achieve. Simpler alternatives for attaining stable long-term transgene expression exist in the *ex vivo* gene therapy approach. In one of the treatment scenarios, transgenes are integrated randomly, e.g. using lentiviral vectors or naked DNA vectors. It is then possible to select the best clone with minimal initial transgene silencing and minimal propensity for transgene expression shutdown among a heterogeneous population of transfected or transduced cells. The preferred method for cell selection is antibody-based magnetic sorting, as this method allows processing of large numbers of cells without recourse to heterologous fluorescent proteins and mutagenic UV irradiation as in fluorescence activated cell sorting (FACS). Clearly, such a clone pre-selection strategy can be used in conjunction with some other counter-silencing strategies (e.g. multiple random transgene insertions or top-up transgene administrations).

## 4.10. Small molecule enhancers of transgene expression

It is extremely attractive to use small molecule compounds to counteract transgene silencing. Substances known to influence chromatin's state are prime candidates for this role. Thus, histon deacetylase inhibitors Trichostatin A, 4-phenylbutyric acid, butyric acid, valeric acid and caproic acid were successfully used to enhance transgene expression after transient trasfection [66]. Available data indicate that another histone deacetylase inhibitor, valproic acid, and also retinoic acid, which is known to act through a receptor-mediated mechanism, are epigenetically active substances and, therefore, in certain situations could be considered for use as transgene expression stimulants. Some small molecule enhancers could be specific for particular vectors used for gene transfer. Thus, hydroxyurea is known to boost transgene expression after delivery with AAV vectors [67]. In this case, transgene expression is likely to be spurred not through the inhibition of standard silencing mechanisms but rather through the more active synthesis of the second DNA strand in the delivered single-stranded AAV vector DNA [67].

### 4.11. Selection of low immunogenic vectors and transgene products

The elimination of therapeutic gene vectors and transgenic cells by the immune system can imitate the silencing of transgene expression. Thus, the employment of low-immunogenic vectors is a preferred option. Vectors' epitopes should mimic the native epitopes of individual patients and do not match their pre-existing immune profile. Coating vector particles with immunologically inert polymers like polyethyleneglycol is one of the strategies to escape immune surveillance. Alternatively, vector particles can be developed, which are able to mimic the immune-evasion strategy of some viruses that are capable of 'hiding' at the cell surface [68]. Non-immunogenic transgene products, e.g. exclusively human versions of proteins, should be chosen to prevent cell elimination via immune reactions *in vivo*. If required, transgene products should be re-engineered to achieve the 'stealth effect' and to tailor them to the immunological profiles of individual patients.

# 5. Conclusion

Epigenetic control by the target cells can result in permanent transgene silencing or in the instability of transgene expression. Thus, one needs to pursue therapeutic strategies, which can achieve long-term transgene expression by taking advantage of, circumventing or overriding silencing favouritism of the resident gene expression control mechanisms.

There are many levels at which the longevity of transgene expression can be addressed through the gene vector choice, design and administration regimen, including: 1) employment of non-nuclear vectors, e.g. mRNA or Sendai virus based vectors; 2) control of transgene modules' amenity to methylation (e.g. purposeful exclusion of methylation-prone CpG islands); 3) employment of minimised DNA vectors such as minicircle DNA to avoid transgene silencing by the bacterial portion of the plasmid vectors; 4) choice of a suitable promoter-enhancer combination with the judicious use of tissue specific, inducible and ubiquitous promoters; 5) achieving a high number of randomly integrated transgenes; 6) control of the chromosomal integration sites via artificial site-preferences of retroviral integrases, transposases or via harnessing of site-specific integration systems; 7) localisation of transgenes on nuclear episomes; 8) chromatin re-modelling control via *cis*-acting elements such as insulator elements and other LCRs; 9) repeated vector administration; 10) selection of individual cell clones with transgenes integrated into favourable loci; 11) use of chemical reagents influencing the epigenetic state to achieve higher and more long-term transgene expression; and 12) choice of non-immunogenic transgene products to prevent the elimination of transgenic cells via immune reactions *in vivo*.

Clearly, the future solutions to transgene silencing enabling stable long-term expression of therapeutic transgenes will depend on the determined implementation of the above strategies and their effective combinations.

## Author details

Oleg E. Tolmachov[1*], Tatiana Subkhankulova[2] and Tanya Tolmachova[2]

*Address all correspondence to: 125317@live.smuc.ac.uk

1 St. Mary's University College, Twickenham, UK

2 National Heart and Lung Institute, Imperial College London, London, UK

## References

[1] Eissenberg JC: Position effect variegation in drosophila: Towards a genetics of chromatin assembly. Bioessays (1989) 11(1):14-17.

[2] Dion V, Lin Y, Hubert L, Jr., Waterland RA, Wilson JH: Dnmt1 deficiency promotes cag repeat expansion in the mouse germline. Hum Mol Genet (2008) 17(9):1306-1317.

[3] Zaegel V, Guermann B, Le Ret M, Andres C, Meyer D, Erhardt M, Canaday J, Gualberto JM, Imbault P: The plant-specific ssdna binding protein osb1 is involved in the stoichiometric transmission of mitochondrial DNA in arabidopsis. Plant Cell (2006) 18(12):3548-3563.

[4] Kiwaki K, Kanegae Y, Saito I, Komaki S, Nakamura K, Miyazaki JI, Endo F, Matsuda I: Correction of ornithine transcarbamylase deficiency in adult spf(ash) mice and in otc-deficient human hepatocytes with recombinant adenoviruses bearing the cag promoter. Hum Gene Ther (1996) 7(7):821-830.

[5] Thum T, Catalucci D, Bauersachs J: Micrornas: Novel regulators in cardiac development and disease. Cardiovasc Res (2008) 79(4):562-570.

[6] Yao S, Sukonnik T, Kean T, Bharadwaj RR, Pasceri P, Ellis J: Retrovirus silencing, variegation, extinction, and memory are controlled by a dynamic interplay of multiple epigenetic modifications. Mol Ther (2004) 10(1):27-36.

[7] Heard E, Colot V: Chromosome structural proteins and rna-mediated epigenetic silencing. Dev Cell (2008) 14(6):813-814.

[8] Okamoto I, Heard E: The dynamics of imprinted x inactivation during preimplantation development in mice. Cytogenet Genome Res (2006) 113(1-4):318-324.

[9] Blewitt ME, Gendrel AV, Pang Z, Sparrow DB, Whitelaw N, Craig JM, Apedaile A, Hilton DJ, Dunwoodie SL, Brockdorff N, Kay GF et al: Smchd1, containing a structural-maintenance-of-chromosomes hinge domain, has a critical role in x inactivation. Nat Genet (2008) 40(5):663-669.

[10] Williams A, Harker N, Ktistaki E, Veiga-Fernandes H, Roderick K, Tolaini M, Norton T, Williams K, Kioussis D: Position effect variegation and imprinting of transgenes in lymphocytes. Nucleic Acids Res (2008) 36(7):2320-2329.

[11] Festenstein R, Tolaini M, Corbella P, Mamalaki C, Parrington J, Fox M, Miliou A, Jones M, Kioussis D: Locus control region function and heterochromatin-induced position effect variegation. Science (1996) 271(5252):1123-1125.

[12] Hiragami-Hamada K, Xie SQ, Saveliev A, Uribe-Lewis S, Pombo A, Festenstein R: The molecular basis for stability of heterochromatin-mediated silencing in mammals. Epigenetics Chromatin (2009) 2(1):14.

[13] Ashe A, Morgan DK, Whitelaw NC, Bruxner TJ, Vickaryous NK, Cox LL, Butterfield NC, Wicking C, Blewitt ME, Wilkins SJ, Anderson GJ et al: A genome-wide screen for modifiers of transgene variegation identifies genes with critical roles in development. Genome Biol (2008) 9(12):R182.

[14] Pietersen AM, van Lohuizen M: Stem cell regulation by polycomb repressors: Postponing commitment. Curr Opin Cell Biol (2008) 20(2):201-207.

[15] Conerly ML, MacQuarrie KL, Fong AP, Yao Z, Tapscott SJ: Polycomb-mediated repression during terminal differentiation: What don't you want to be when you grow up? Genes Dev (2011) 25(10):997-1003.

[16] Klauke K, de Haan G: Polycomb group proteins in hematopoietic stem cell aging and malignancies. Int J Hematol (2011) 94(1):11-23.

[17] Majewski IJ, Blewitt ME, de Graaf CA, McManus EJ, Bahlo M, Hilton AA, Hyland CD, Smyth GK, Corbin JE, Metcalf D, Alexander WS et al: Polycomb repressive complex 2 (prc2) restricts hematopoietic stem cell activity. PLoS Biol (2008) 6(4):e93.

[18] Sawarkar R, Paro R: Interpretation of developmental signaling at chromatin: The polycomb perspective. Dev Cell (2010) 19(5):651-661.

[19] Leeb C, Jurga M, McGuckin C, Forraz N, Thallinger C, Moriggl R, Kenner L: New perspectives in stem cell research: Beyond embryonic stem cells. Cell Prolif (2011) 44 Suppl 1(9-14.

[20] Petruk S, Sedkov Y, Riley KM, Hodgson J, Schweisguth F, Hirose S, Jaynes JB, Brock HW, Mazo A: Transcription of bxd noncoding rnas promoted by trithorax represses ubx in cis by transcriptional interference. Cell (2006) 127(6):1209-1221.

[21] Sanchez-Elsner T, Gou D, Kremmer E, Sauer F: Noncoding rnas of trithorax response elements recruit drosophila ash1 to ultrabithorax. Science (2006) 311(5764):1118-1123.

[22]  Schmidt FR: About the nature of rna interference. Applied microbiology and biotech-nology (2005) 67(4):429-435.

[23]  Zentilin L, Qin G, Tafuro S, Dinauer MC, Baum C, Giacca M: Variegation of retrovi-ral vector gene expression in myeloid cells. Gene Ther (2000) 7(2):153-166.

[24]  Dorer DR, Henikoff S: Expansions of transgene repeats cause heterochromatin for-mation and gene silencing in drosophila. Cell (1994) 77(7):993-1002.

[25]  Saveliev A, Everett C, Sharpe T, Webster Z, Festenstein R: DNA triplet repeats medi-ate heterochromatin-protein-1-sensitive variegated gene silencing. Nature (2003) 422(6934):909-913.

[26]  Cao B, Bruder J, Kovesdi I, Huard J: Muscle stem cells can act as antigen-presenting cells: Implication for gene therapy. Gene Ther (2004) 11(17):1321-1330.

[27]  Chen ZY, He CY, Meuse L, Kay MA: Silencing of episomal transgene expression by plasmid bacterial DNA elements in vivo. Gene Ther (2004) 11(10):856-864.

[28]  Suzuki M, Kasai K, Saeki Y: Plasmid DNA sequences present in conventional herpes simplex virus amplicon vectors cause rapid transgene silencing by forming inactive chromatin. J Virol (2006) 80(7):3293-3300.

[29]  Chen ZY, Riu E, He CY, Xu H, Kay MA: Silencing of episomal transgene expression in liver by plasmid bacterial backbone DNA is independent of cpg methylation. Mol Ther (2008) 16(3):548-556.

[30]  McLachlan G, Stevenson BJ, Davidson DJ, Porteous DJ: Bacterial DNA is implicated in the inflammatory response to delivery of DNA/dotap to mouse lungs. Gene Ther (2000) 7(5):384-392.

[31]  Butash KA, Natarajan P, Young A, Fox DK: Reexamination of the effect of endotoxin on cell proliferation and transfection efficiency. Biotechniques (2000) 29(3):610-614, 616, 618-619.

[32]  Weber M, Moller K, Welzeck M, Schorr J: Short technical reports. Effects of lipopoly-saccharide on transfection efficiency in eukaryotic cells. Biotechniques (1995) 19(6): 930-940.

[33]  Arenas J: The role of bacterial lipopolysaccharides as immune modulator in vaccine and drug development. Endocrine, metabolic & immune disorders drug targets (2012) 12(3):221-235.

[34]  Kuhn AN, Beissert T, Simon P, Vallazza B, Buck J, Davies BP, Tureci O, Sahin U: Mrna as a versatile tool for exogenous protein expression. Curr Gene Ther (2012).

[35]  Zhang Q, Li Y, Shi Y, Zhang Y: Hvj envelope vector, a versatile delivery system: Its development, application, and perspectives. Biochem Biophys Res Commun (2008) 373(3):345-349.

[36] Marie C, Vandermeulen G, Quiviger M, Richard M, Preat V, Scherman D: Pfars, plasmids free of antibiotic resistance markers, display high-level transgene expression in muscle, skin and tumour cells. J Gene Med (2010) 12(4):323-332.

[37] Mairhofer J, Grabherr R: Rational vector design for efficient non-viral gene delivery: Challenges facing the use of plasmid DNA. Molecular biotechnology (2008) 39(2): 97-104.

[38] Hirata K, Nishikawa M, Kobayashi N, Takahashi Y, Takakura Y: Design of pcr-amplified DNA fragments for in vivo gene delivery: Size-dependency on stability and transgene expression. J Pharm Sci (2007) 96(9):2251-2261.

[39] Schakowski F, Gorschluter M, Buttgereit P, Marten A, Lilienfeld-Toal MV, Junghans C, Schroff M, Konig-Merediz SA, Ziske C, Strehl J, Sauerbruch T et al: Minimal size midge vectors improve transgene expression in vivo. In Vivo (2007) 21(1):17-23.

[40] Bigger BW, Tolmachov O, Collombet JM, Fragkos M, Palaszewski I, Coutelle C: An arac-controlled bacterial cre expression system to produce DNA minicircle vectors for nuclear and mitochondrial gene therapy. J Biol Chem (2001) 276(25):23018-23027.

[41] Argyros O, Wong SP, Fedonidis C, Tolmachov O, Waddington SN, Howe SJ, Niceta M, Coutelle C, Harbottle RP: Development of s/mar minicircles for enhanced and persistent transgene expression in the mouse liver. J Mol Med (2011) 89(5):515-529.

[42] Zhao N, Fogg JM, Zechiedrich L, Zu Y: Transfection of shrna-encoding minivector DNA of a few hundred base pairs to regulate gene expression in lymphoma cells. Gene Ther (2011) 18(3):220-224.

[43] Hong S, Hwang DY, Yoon S, Isacson O, Ramezani A, Hawley RG, Kim KS: Functional analysis of various promoters in lentiviral vectors at different stages of in vitro differentiation of mouse embryonic stem cells. Mol Ther (2007) 15(9):1630-1639.

[44] Tolmachova T, Tolmachov OE, Wavre-Shapton ST, Tracey-White D, Futter CE, Seabra MC: Chm/rep1 cdna delivery by lentiviral vectors provides functional expression of the transgene in the retinal pigment epithelium of choroideremia mice. J Gene Med (2012) 14(3):158-168.

[45] Papadakis ED, Nicklin SA, Baker AH, White SJ: Promoters and control elements: Designing expression cassettes for gene therapy. Curr Gene Ther (2004) 4(1):89-113.

[46] Tolmachov OE: Building mosaics of therapeutic plasmid gene vectors. Curr Gene Ther (2011) 11(6):466-478.

[47] Huang X, Guo H, Tammana S, Jung YC, Mellgren E, Bassi P, Cao Q, Tu ZJ, Kim YC, Ekker SC, Wu X et al: Gene transfer efficiency and genome-wide integration profiling of sleeping beauty, tol2, and piggybac transposons in human primary t cells. Mol Ther (2010) 18(10):1803-1813.

[48] Yant SR, Huang Y, Akache B, Kay MA: Site-directed transposon integration in human cells. Nucleic Acids Res (2007) 35(7):e50.

[49] Keravala A, Lee S, Thyagarajan B, Olivares EC, Gabrovsky VE, Woodard LE, Calos MP: Mutational derivatives of phic31 integrase with increased efficiency and specificity. Mol Ther (2009) 17(1):112-120.

[50] Thomson JG, Ow DW: Site-specific recombination systems for the genetic manipulation of eukaryotic genomes. Genesis (2006) 44(10):465-476.

[51] Huang S, Kawabe Y, Ito A, Kamihira M: Adeno-associated virus rep-mediated targeting of integrase-defective retroviral vector DNA circles into human chromosome 19. Biochem Biophys Res Commun (2012) 417(1):78-83.

[52] Howden SE, Voullaire L, Vadolas J: The transient expression of mrna coding for rep protein from aav facilitates targeted plasmid integration. J Gene Med (2008) 10(1): 42-50.

[53] Humme S, Reisbach G, Feederle R, Delecluse HJ, Bousset K, Hammerschmidt W, Schepers A: The ebv nuclear antigen 1 (ebna1) enhances b cell immortalization several thousandfold. Proc Natl Acad Sci U S A (2003) 100(19):10989-10994.

[54] Hagedorn C, Wong SP, Harbottle R, Lipps HJ: Scaffold/matrix attached region-based nonviral episomal vectors. Hum Gene Ther (2011) 22(8):915-923.

[55] Rangasamy D: An s/mar-based l1 retrotransposition cassette mediates sustained levels of insertional mutagenesis without suffering from epigenetic silencing of DNA methylation. Epigenetics 5(7):601-611.

[56] Broll S, Oumard A, Hahn K, Schambach A, Bode J: Minicircle performance depending on s/mar-nuclear matrix interactions. J Mol Biol 395(5):950-965.

[57] Bunnell BA, Izadpanah R, Ledebur Jr HC, Perez CF: Development of mammalian artificial chromosomes for the treatment of genetic diseases: Sandhoff and krabbe diseases. Expert Opin Biol Ther (2005) 5(2):195-206.

[58] Macnab S, Whitehouse A: Progress and prospects: Human artificial chromosomes. Gene Ther (2009) 16(10):1180-1188.

[59] Macarthur CC, Xue H, Van Hoof D, Lieu PT, Dudas M, Fontes A, Swistowski A, Touboul T, Seerke R, Laurent LC, Loring JF et al: Chromatin insulator elements block transgene silencing in engineered human embryonic stem cell lines at a defined chromosome 13 locus. Stem cells and development (2012) 21(2):191-205.

[60] Li Q, Harju S, Peterson KR: Locus control regions: Coming of age at a decade plus. Trends Genet (1999) 15(10):403-408.

[61] Lee GR, Fields PE, Griffin TJ, Flavell RA: Regulation of the th2 cytokine locus by a locus control region. Immunity (2003) 19(1):145-153.

[62] Nielsen TT, Jakobsson J, Rosenqvist N, Lundberg C: Incorporating double copies of a chromatin insulator into lentiviral vectors results in less viral integrants. BMC Biotechnol (2009) 9(13.

[63] Grandchamp N, Henriot D, Philippe S, Amar L, Ursulet S, Serguera C, Mallet J, Sarkis C: Influence of insulators on transgene expression from integrating and non-integrating lentiviral vectors. Genet Vaccines Ther 9(1):1.

[64] Wang F, Wang TY, Tang YY, Zhang JH, Yang XJ: Different matrix attachment regions flanking a transgene effectively enhance gene expression in stably transfected chinese hamster ovary cells. Gene (2012) 500(1):59-62.

[65] Harraghy N, Gaussin A, Mermod N: Sustained transgene expression using mar elements. Curr Gene Ther (2008) 8(5):353-366.

[66] Nan X, Hyndman L, Agbi N, Porteous DJ, Boyd AC: Potent stimulation of gene expression by histone deacetylase inhibitors on transiently transfected DNA. Biochem Biophys Res Commun (2004) 324(1):348-354.

[67] Ju XD, Lou SQ, Wang WG, Peng JQ, Tian H: Effect of hydroxyurea and etoposide on transduction of human bone marrow mesenchymal stem and progenitor cell by adeno-associated virus vectors. Acta pharmacologica Sinica (2004) 25(2):196-202.

[68] Ilett EJ, Barcena M, Errington-Mais F, Griffin S, Harrington KJ, Pandha HS, Coffey M, Selby PJ, Limpens RW, Mommaas M, Hoeben RC et al: Internalization of oncolytic reovirus by human dendritic cell carriers protects the virus from neutralization. Clin Cancer Res (2011) 17(9):2767-2776.

# Chapter 3

# Plasmid Transgene Expression *in vivo*: Promoter and Tissue Variables

David Morrissey, Sara A. Collins, Simon Rajenderan,
Garrett Casey, Gerald C. O'Sullivan and
Mark Tangney

Additional information is available at the end of the chapter

## 1. Introduction

Ensuring an appropriate level and duration of expression is essential in achieving an efficient and safe gene therapy. While the length of time a gene must be expressed for efficacy
depends on both the therapeutic strategy and the disease, many gene therapy approaches
prove ineffective as the therapeutic is expressed for a limited duration (Frank et al. 2004).
Proposed causes of transient expression include loss of DNA due to cell turnover, immune
responses against transfected cells and/or expressed proteins, and inhibition of transcription
through host cell methylation of microbial DNA sequences (Prosch et al. 1996; Scheule 2000;
Greenland et al. 2007). Vector related elements or activity also contribute to duration of gene
expression post administration. Adenovirus is known to stimulate severe innate and adaptive immune responses, and can induce cellular and humoural responses to the transgene
product and its capsid proteins resulting in failure to provide long-term gene expression
(Jooss et al. 1998; Yuasa et al. 2002; Louboutin et al. 2005; Wang et al. 2005).

Plasmid electroporation, on the other hand, has been shown not to elicit such transgene
gene silencing immune responses (Jooss et al. 1998; Mir et al. 1999), and presents an attractive option in achieving long-term gene expression, especially in light of recent improve-
ments in plasmid vectors (Gill et al. 2009). Although plasmid based systems offer certain
advantages, they do, however, have drawbacks. The magnitude of transgene expression is
generally lower with plasmid vectors than that with viruses. In addition, most plasmids are
not passed on to daughter cells following cell division leading to eventual loss of expression
in rapidly dividing tissues. This can result in sub-therapeutic effects, a significant problem

with gene therapy. Efforts have been made to ensure that therapeutic protein production is active for an appropriate length of time to address some of these failings. To counteract the effects of episomal DNA loss, the use of integrating DNA in the form of retroviruses or transposon containing plasmids has been examined and shown some efficacy(Sandrin et al. 2003; Ohlfest et al. 2005). Delivery in this fashion would lead to long lasting, possibly indefinite gene expression. Although this addresses one failing of plasmid delivery, the potential of indefinite and uncontrollable protein production to cause unexpected side effects is an issue. Unlike the current situation, where therapy related complications results in withdrawal of the medication, the "offending gene" cannot easily be removed, and may continue to cause significant side effects. In addition, integration of foreign DNA is not ideal as it can lead to mutagenesis, with subsequent alteration in the patient's protein expression profile and potentially carcinogenesis. With this in mind, methods of prolonging and/or controlling episomal gene expression are preferred, provided this expression is of sufficient magnitude.

Plasmid loss alone may not fully account for the temporal loss of expression seen with these vectors. Epigenetic modification of the therapeutic has also been implicated in gene silencing, but the exact mechanisms by which this occurs have not yet been fully elucidated. It has been demonstrated that duration of transgene expression may by increased by use of 'native' promoters of mammalian origin rather than viral promoters (Gazdhar et al. 2006). The postulated mechanism behind this difference of expression relates to the presence and subsequent methylation of CpG sequences on promoters. This methylation is a naturally occurring phenomenon and reports have correlated methylation of CpG-rich sequences with silencing of gene expression (Gazdhar, Bilici et al. 2006). Native mammalian promoters possess fewer CpG sequences than their viral counterparts and are theoretically less prone to silencing. By employing mammalian promoters, the duration of gene expression may be extended, allowing for sustained therapeutic production. Anecdotal evidence suggests that the degree of viral promoter silencing varies between tissue types, and that the duration of gene expression in tumour tissue in particular may be short-lived (Jaenisch et al. 1985; Momparler & Bovenzi 2000; Bartoli et al. 2003). This may, in part, be due to abnormal cell turnover in tumour tissue, but the disorganised methylation pattern in tumour tissue could also play a role.

In this chapter, we assess the influence of promoter type on electroporated plasmid transgene expression in murine models. Expression is examined by utilising the reporter gene luciferase. The activity of luciferase can then be measured *in vivo*, allowing for repeated assessment of gene expression in the same test subjects over time. The pattern of expression is also examined in different tissue types as is the role of epigenetic modification in gene silencing.

## 2. Materials and methods

### 2.1. DNA constructs

pGL3-Control and pCMV-luc were purchased from Stratagene (Techno-Path, Limerick, Ireland) and Promega (Medical Supply Co., Dublin, Ireland) respectively. pDRIVE03-UbiquitinB(h) v02 was purchased from Invivogen (Cayla SAS, Toulouse, France). A version of this plasmid, designated pUb-luc, containing the firefly *luciferase* gene transcriptionally controlled from the human Ubiquitin-B promoter was constructed, by excising the firefly *luciferase* gene from pGL3-Control using restriction enzymes Nco1 and Xba1 (New England Biolabs, USA) and cloning it in the Nhe1 (site 2) and Nco1 sites of pDRIVE03-UbiquitinB(h) downstream of the ubiquitin promoter. Plasmid copy number was calculated using the formula number DNA copies = weight/(Plasmid size x $1.096$ x $10^{-21}$) with pUb-luc = $4.3$ x$10^3$, pCMV-luc = $5.9$ x $10^3$ and pGL3 = $5.2$ x $10^3$ bp respectively. Endotoxin-free plasmid DNA was isolated from TOP10F *E.coli* (Invitrogen) using the MegaPrep kit (Qiagen, West Sussex, England).

## 2.2. Animals and tumour induction

Murine JBS fibrosarcoma tumour cells were maintained in culture in Dulbecco's Modified Essential Medium (DMEM) (GIBCO, Invitrogen Corp., Paisley, Scotland) as previously described (Collins, C. G. et al. 2006; Collins, S. A. et al. 2010). Female Balb/C and MF1nu/nu mice of 6–8 weeks of age were obtained from Harlan Laboratories (Oxfordshire, England). For routine tumour induction, $2 \times 10^6$ JBS cells suspended in 200 µl serum free DMEM were injected subcutaneously into the flank.

## 2.3. *In-vivo* gene delivery

For tumour experiments, mice were treated at a tumour volume of approximately 100 mm³ in volume (5-7 mm major diameter). Mice were anaesthetized during all treatments by intraperitoneal (i.p.) administration of 200 µg xylazine and 2 mg ketamine. For liver transfection, a 1 cm subcostal incision was made over the liver and the peritoneum opened. The right lobe of the exposed liver was administered plasmid by electroporation as described below (Casey et al. 2010; Collins, S. A. et al. 2011). The wound was closed in two layers, peritoneal and skin, using 4/0 prolene sutures (Promed, Killorglin, Ireland). For plasmid delivery by electroporation, a custom-designed applicator with 2 needles 4 mm apart was used, with both needles placed through the skin central to the tissue. Tissue was injected between electrode needles with $8$ x $10^{11}$ copies of plasmid DNA in sterile injectable saline in an injection volume of 50 µl. After 80 seconds, square-wave pulses (1200 V/cm 100 µsec x 1 and 120 V/cm 20 msec, 8 pulses) were administered in sequence using a custom designed pulse generator (Cliniporator (IGEA, Carpi, Italy).

## 2.4. Inhibition of DNA acetylation *in vivo*

Individual animals were weighed and dosed by i.p. injection of trichostatin A (TSA) (Sigma) at 10 mg/kg in 60 µl 10% (v/v) dimethyl sulfoxide in filtered peanut oil, daily for the duration of the experiment. *In vivo* luciferase activity was assessed 4 hours after administration of TSA.

## 2.5. Whole body imaging

*In vivo* luciferase activity from tissues was analysed at set time points post-transfection as follows: 80 µl of 30 mg/ml firefly luciferin (Biosynth, Basil, Switzerland) was injected i.p.

and intratumourally where appropriate. Mice were anaesthetised as before. Ten minutes post-luciferin injection, live anaesthetised mice were imaged for 3 min at high sensitivity using an intensified CCD camera (IVIS Imaging System, Xenogen, Caliper Life Sciences, England). Exposure conditions were maintained at identical levels so that all measurements would be comparable. All data analysis was carried out on Living Image 2.5 software (Xenogen). Luminescence levels were calculated using standardised regions of interest (ROI) for all three anatomical areas. Actual levels were obtained by subtracting the corresponding ROI of an untransfected mouse to account for background luminescence. For comparison between plasmids, luminescence was represented as $p/sec/cm^2/sr/plasmid$ copy.

### 2.6. Assessment of plasmid DNA in liver tissue using PCR analysis

To determine the presence of plasmid DNA in liver tissue, pCMV-Luc was delivered to the livers of 9 mice using electroporation as previously described. Luciferase expression was assessed by IVIS imaging at the time of sampling, 24 hr, 3 days and 10 days post treatment. Livers from three mice were excised at each time-point and snap frozen in liquid nitrogen. Livers were homogenized in TRIZOL Reagent (Invitrogen) using an Ultra Turrax T25 homogeniser (IKA Werke GmbH & Co. KG, Staufen, Germany) and total DNA was extracted as per the manufacturer's protocol. The presence of the plasmid DNA in the total DNA was determined by PCR using *luciferase* specific primers (For- 5′-AATCCATCTTGCTCCAA-CAC-3′ Rev- 5′ATCTCTTTTTCCGTCATCGTC-3′). PCR conditions were: Initial denaturation at 95 ºC for 15mins followed by 35 cycles (95 ºC for 1 min, 60 ºC for 1 min, 72 ºC for 1 min) and a final extension of 10 m at 72 ºC. The resulting PCR products were analyzed on a 1 % agarose gel.

### 2.7. Statistical analysis

The primary outcome variable of the statistical analyses was luminescence per cell per gene copy administered in each cell line or luminescence per gene copy administered in each organ measured at each time point. The principal explanatory variables were the delivery modalites used. *In vivo* luminescence was analysed as continuous. At specified time points, a two-sampled t-test was used to compare mean luminescence per gene copy administered for each delivery modality. Microsoft Excel 11.0 (Microsoft) and GraphPad Prism Version 4.0 (GraphPad Prism Software Inc, San Diego, CA, USA) were used to manage and analyze data. Statistical significance was defined at the standard 5 % level.

## 3. Results

Plasmid DNA encoding the luciferase gene transcribed from either the CMV (pCMV-luc) or Ubiquitin-B (pUb-luc) promoter was delivered to murine liver or quadriceps muscle by *in vivo* electroporation. Live whole body imaging (IVIS) was performed at various times over 370 days to determine luciferase expression. Expression mediated by the CMV promoter in liver, while initially high, reduced rapidly to background level by day 7 (figure 1a). When the Ub promoter plasmid was examined in livers (figure 1b), luminescence was initially low but increased during the first week post transfection, before decreasing slowly, and remained higher than the CMV levels up to day 25. To examine other viral promoter activity in liver, pGL3 (SV40 promoter) was assessed (figure 1c). Like pCMV-luc, pGL3 displayed significantly faster reduction in expression than pUb-luc. A different temporal pattern of expression was observed in muscle for both the CMV and Ub promoters. Although promoter activity fluctuated over the period examined, a gross reduction in expression over time was not observed in this tissue with either CMV or Ub promoters (figure 1).

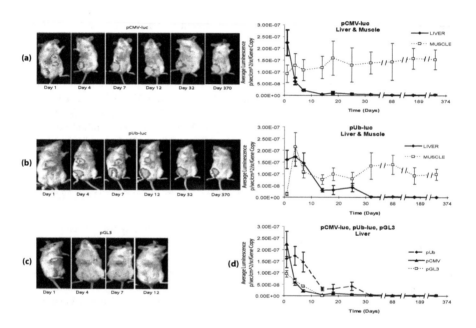

**Figure 1. Duration of CMV and Ub promoter activity *in vivo* in liver and muscle** pCMV-luc, pUb-luc or pGL3 was delivered to liver and quadriceps muscle (n=8) by electroporation and luminescence analysed *in vivo* over time using IVIS imaging. **(a)** CMV activity in liver was initially high, reducing to background levels by day 7. **(b)** Initial Ub activity levels were lower than those detected for the CMV promoter but increased and remained higher than that detected for CMV at later time points up to day 25. A gross reduction in expression over time was not apparent in muscle with either CMV or Ub promoters. **(c)** SV40 expression in liver decreased to background levels by Day 7. **(d)** Expression levels from both viral promoters (CMV and SV40) decline significantly faster than Ub in liver.

The kinetics of CMV, Ub and SV40 promoter activity were also analysed in tumour bearing mice. pCMV-luc, pUb-luc or pGL3 DNA was electroporated to subcutaneous (s.c.) JBS fibrosarcoma tumours upon reaching 80 mm³ in volume. IVIS imaging over 18 days (the limit of tumour monitoring before animals required culling) demonstrated that the initially high expression driven by the CMV promoter was rapidly reduced to background level by day 4-post transfection (figure 2). Reduction was also observed with SV40 promoter, albeit with a heterologous temporal expression pattern to CMV, with pGL3 expression peaking at day 4 before rapidly reducing to background levels. Ub promoter activity was still evident at the final time point. pCMV-luc and pGL3 displayed statistically similar (p = 0.98) maximum to minimum rates of silencing ($2.9 \times 10^{-7}$ p/sec/cm$^2$/sr/gene copy per day), higher than that of pUb-luc ($6.8 \times 10^{-8}$ p/sec/cm$^2$/sr/gene copy per day). pCMV-luc expression was also found to rapidly reduce in s.c. human MCF7 breast carcinoma tumours growing in athymic mice (data not shown). Ubiquitin-B promoter transcriptional activity may be related to the normal functions of ubiquitin in cells, which is expressed constitutively for removing abnormal proteins and for modification of histones leading to gene activation, and so may not be subject to the down-regulation observed with many viral promoters (Ciechanover et al. 2000; Yew et al. 2001). Ubiquitin is also induced in response to cell stress, and expression might be up-regulated in response to cellular necrosis and apoptosis, which is especially relevant in growing tumours. Given that pUb-luc expression is evident long after viral promoter activity diminishes (up to day 25 for pUb-luc as opposed to day 7 for pCMV-luc and pGL3; figure 2), it is plausible that viral promoter plasmids remain present in liver post cessation of expression.

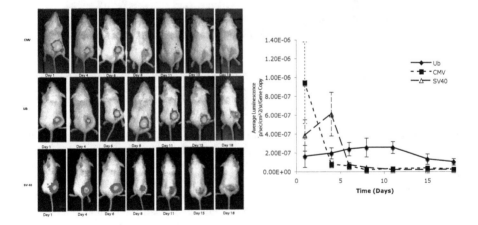

**Figure 2. Duration of viral and native promoter activity in tumour** pCMV-luc, pGL3 or pUb-luc was delivered *in vivo* to growing tumours (n=6) by electroporation and luminescence analysed *in vivo* over time using IVIS imaging. Expression from both viral promoters (CMV and SV40) rapidly diminished, whereas Ub promoter activity was still evident at the final time point (day 18) when mice required culling due to tumour size. Ub mediated expression levels were at 39.4 % of maximal level on final time-point, compared with 2.4 % and 3.5 % for CMV and SV40 respectively.

To test for the presence of plasmid, DNA was extracted from murine livers at various times post transfection with pCMV-luc and PCR analysis performed. DNA PCR results from days 1, 3 and 10 confirmed the presence of *luciferase* DNA in tissue after cessation of expression, suggesting that inhibition of transgene expression occurred at the level of or post transcription (figure 3). Our findings indicate that both viral promoters examined provided short-lived expression in tumours and liver, whereas use of Ub promoter significantly prolonged transgene expression. Importantly, we also found that viral promoter activity was dependent on target tissue, since no reduction in expression was observed in plasmid electroporated muscle with both viral and mammalian promoters.

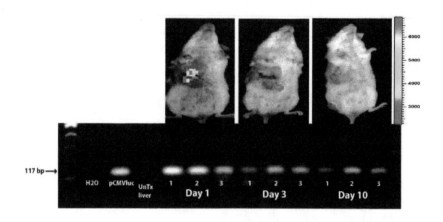

**Figure 3. Plasmid DNA persists in liver after cessation of expression** PCR analysis of DNA extracted from murine livers (n=3) on days 1, 3 or 10-post electroporation with pCMV-luc. A representative mouse from which DNA was extracted at each time-point is shown. PCR using primers specific for the *luciferase* gene indicates presence of plasmid. Untransfected liver samples did not yield PCR product.

In order to examine any effects of T-cell mediated immune activity on viral promoter construct expression, pCMV-luc expression in livers of athymic mice was examined. No difference in the magnitude or duration of expression was observed between immune competent Balb/C and T-cell deficient mice, suggesting that cellular immune responses were not involved in the observed reduction in hepatic expression of pCMV-luc (figure 4a). Other studies have indicated that luciferase protein has low immunogenicity, and immune-mediated destruction of luciferase-producing cells does not occur in mice (Davis et al. 1997), while the persistence of expression in muscle here also makes this unlikely as a cause for silencing in other tissues. The observation of indefinite expression in plasmid electroporated muscle is in direct contrast to Ad expression in quadriceps muscle, which has been shown to be eliminated through T cell and antibody immune activities and/or CMV promoter methylation (Jooss, Yang et al. 1998; Brooks et al. 2004).

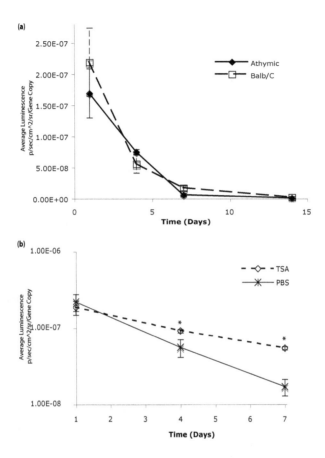

**Figure 4. (a) pCMV-luc is silenced in livers in absence of T cells** pCMV-luc was electroporated *in vivo* to livers of athymic mice and IVIS imaged (n=4). No difference was observed in plasmid expression at any time point when compared with expression in immunocompetent Balb/C mice (p > 0.25). **(b) Effect of deacetylation agent on pCMV-luc expression *in vivo*** pCMV-luc was delivered to livers by electroporation (n=4). TSA or PBS was i.p. administered daily. Gene expression was analysed using the IVIS imaging system. The magnitude and duration of gene expression in animals treated with TSA was significantly increased. * denotes statistically significant difference between groups, p < 0.05.

## 4. Discussion

We did not determine the reasons for the observed tissue-specific nature of viral promoter silencing, and it remains unclear as to why liver and tumour, but not muscle, affected plasmid expression. Plasmids function predominantly in an episomal fashion and copy number per cell is reduced proportional to cell replication. As such, genes would be expected to be diluted rapidly in tissues with a high mitotic index. Liver hepatocytes and skeletal myocytes are fully differentiated and have a low turnover, unlike tumour cells. (Ayers & Jeffery 1988) It may be hypothesised that the static nature of cell turnover in muscle compared with tumour is relevant in this context. However, this cannot fully account for the observed loss of expression, since in our study, the rate of reduction of expression for plasmids with promoters of mammalian and viral origin was different. Also, previous studies have shown no alteration in longevity of transgene expression when cell turnover was inhibited (Herweijer et al. 2001). Furthermore, we demonstrated by PCR that pCMV-luc persisted in liver cells after expression ceased. We think it is unlikely that the reduction in pCMV-luc expression was due to a parallel reduction in the plasmid DNA as this was not seen for the Ub promoter where similar plasmid copy numbers would be expected.

It has previously been demonstrated that plasmid transgene expression can be modulated with chromatin remodelling agents (Bartoli, Fettucciari et al. 2003). To this end, murine livers were electroporated with pCMV-luc and mice systemically administered the histone deacetylase inhibitor trichostatin-A (TSA) daily for the duration of experiment. TSA is a specific inhibitor for histone deacetylase (HDAC) and is known to enhance gene expression in viral and plasmid-transfected cells *in vitro* and *in vivo* (Vanniasinkam et al. 2006). It has been shown that HDAC binds to the CMV promoter, and TSA may act to overcome such transcriptional repression (Tang & Maul 2003). In our experiments, TSA administration significantly increased levels of expression at later time points, compared with control ($p <$ 0.002 on day 7; figure 4b). Interestingly, a further increase was noted when 5' azacytidine (aza-C), a non-specific methylation inhibitor, and trichostatin were used in combination, while aza-C in isolation had no effect (data not shown).

While this study did not generate data to correlate RNA levels with luminescence, differences in transcription appears to be the key element in observed expression levels. Firefly luciferase protein is known to have a short half-life *in vivo*, in the region of 1 - 4 hours (Baggett et al. 2004; Tangney & Francis 2012), and any luminescence detected in our experiments was due to recently transcribed gene. Furthermore, given that pUb-luc expression is evident long after viral promoter activity diminishes (up to day 25 for pUb-luc as opposed to day 7 for pCMV-luc and pGL3; figure 1), it is likely that viral promoter plasmids remain present in liver post cessation of expression, and we demonstrated by PCR that pCMV-luc DNA was present in liver 10 days post transfection.There exist numerous reports linking viral promoter DNA methylation with transcriptional silencing in gene therapy settings *in vitro* and *in vivo* (Di Ianni et al. 1999; Brooks, Harkins et al. 2004; Al-Dosari et al. 2006).

Our findings are consistent with previous studies in lung tissue where the levels and duration of transgene expression *in vivo* were compared using plasmid vectors coding for the CMV or Ubiquitin promoters (Gill et al. 2001; Yew, Przybylska et al. 2001; Gazdhar, Bilici et al. 2006). Further specific methylation assays may elucidate the precise mechanism of viral promoter silencing here. Given that many tumour types have been shown to have abnormal methylation, this phenomenon may represent a serious hindrance to cancer gene therapy which use of native promoters may abrogate as demonstrated here (Kanai 2008). Furthermore, the finding of indefinite high-level expression in plasmid electroporated muscle irrespective of the promoter type has important therapeutic implications. Skeletal muscle is a large and accessible tissue, within which a plasmid-based gene therapy might be a safe and efficient method for systemic protein production, particularly when combined with either endogenous or exogenous regulatable systems. We have previously demonstrated the application of an inducible plasmid based system in *in vivo* murine tissue (Morrissey et al. 2012). In addition to providing an "off switch" to safeguard against side effects, this also allows optimal temporal delivery of therapeutic, tailored to when it can most efficiently achieve a biological response.

## 5. Conclusion

In summary these results highlight the importance of promoter,tissue and vector variables in achieving appropriate transgene expression for DNA therapeutic strategies.

## Acknowledgment

This work was funded by Cancer Research Ireland (CRI07TAN) and the Cork Cancer Research Centre.

## Author details

David Morrissey, Sara A. Collins, Simon Rajenderan, Garrett Casey, Gerald C. O'Sullivan and Mark Tangney

Cork Cancer Research Centre, Mercy University Hospital and Leslie C. Quick Jnr. Laboratory, University College Cork, Cork, Ireland

## References

[1] Al-Dosari, M., Zhang, G., Knapp, J. E., & Liu, D. (2006). Evaluation of viral and mammalian promoters for driving transgene expression in mouse liver. Biochem Biophys Res Commun , 339(2), 673-8.

[2] Ayers, M. M., & Jeffery, P. K. (1988). Proliferation and differentiation in mammalian airway epithelium. Eur Respir J , 1(1), 58-80.

[3] Baggett, B., Roy, R., Momen, S., Morgan, S., Tisi, L., Morse, D., & Gillies, R. J. (2004). Thermostability of firefly luciferases affects efficiency of detection by in vivo bioluminescence. Mol Imaging , 3(4), 324-32.

[4]   Bartoli, A., Fettucciari, K., Fetriconi, I., Rosati, E., Di Ianni, M., Tabilio, A., Delfino, D. V., Rossi, R., & Marconi, P. (2003). Effect of trichostatin a and 5′-azacytidine on transgene reactivation in U937 transduced cells. Pharmacol Res , 48(1), 111-8.

[5]   Brooks, A. R., Harkins, R. N., Wang, P., Qian, H. S., Liu, P., & Rubanyi, G. M. (2004). Transcriptional silencing is associated with extensive methylation of the CMV promoter following adenoviral gene delivery to muscle. J Gene Med , 6(4), 395-404.

[6]   Casey, G., Cashman, J. P., Morrissey, D., Whelan, M. C., Larkin, J. O., Soden, D. M., Tangney, M., & O'Sullivan, G. C. (2010). Sonoporation mediated immunogene therapy of solid tumors. Ultrasound Med Biol 36(3): X (Electronic)0301-5629 (Linking), 430 EOF-440 EOF.

[7]   Ciechanover, A., Orian, A., & Schwartz, A. L. (2000). Ubiquitin-mediated proteolysis: biological regulation via destruction. Bioessays , 22(5), 442-51.

[8]   Collins, C. G., Tangney, M., Larkin, J. O., Casey, G., Whelan, M. C., Cashman, J., Murphy, J., Soden, D., Vejda, S., Mc Kenna, S., Kiely, B., Collins, J. K., Barrett, J., Aarons, S., & O'Sullivan, G. C. (2006). Local gene therapy of solid tumors with GM-CSF and B71 eradicates both treated and distal tumors. Cancer Gene Ther

[9]   Collins, S. A., Buhles, A., Scallan, M. F., Harrison, P. T., O'Hanlon, D. M., O'Sullivan, G. C., & Tangney, M. (2010). AAV2 -mediated in vivo immune gene therapy of solid tumours. Genet Vaccines Ther 8: 81479-0556 (Electronic)1479-0556 (Linking)

[10]  Collins, S. A., Morrissey, D., Rajendran, S., Casey, G., Scallan, M. F., Harrison, P. T., O'Sullivan, G. C., & Tangney, M. (2011). Comparison of DNA Delivery and Expression Using Frequently Used Delivery Methods. Gene Therapy- developments and future perspectives. C. Kang, InTech.

[11]  Davis, H. L., Millan, C. L., & Watkins, S. C. (1997). Immune-mediated destruction of transfected muscle fibers after direct gene transfer with antigen-expressing plasmid DNA. Gene Ther , 4(3), 181-8.

[12]  Di Ianni, M., Terenzi, A., Perruccio, K., Ciurnelli, R., Lucheroni, F., Benedetti, R., Martelli, M. F., & Tabilio, A. (1999). 5 -Azacytidine prevents transgene methylation in vivo. Gene Ther 6(4): 703-70969-7128 (Print)

[13]  Frank, O., Rudolph, C., Heberlein, C., von, Neuhoff. N., Schrock, E., Schambach, A., Schlegelberger, B., Fehse, B., Ostertag, W., Stocking, C., & Baum, C. (2004). Tumor cells escape suicide gene therapy by genetic and epigenetic instability. *Blood*, 104(12), 3543-9.

[14]  Gazdhar, A., Bilici, M., Pierog, J., Ayuni, E. L., Gugger, M., Wetterwald, A., Cecchini, M., & Schmid, R. A. (2006). In vivo electroporation and ubiquitin promoter- a protocol for sustained gene expression in the lung." J Gene Med , 8(7), 910-918.

[15]  Gill, D. R., Pringle, I. A., & Hyde, S. C. (2009). Progress and prospects: the design and production of plasmid vectors. Gene Ther , 16(2), 165-71.

[16] Gill, D. R., Smyth, S. E., Goddard, C. A., Pringle, I. A., Higgins, C. F., Colledge, W. H., & Hyde, S. C. (2001). Increased persistence of lung gene expression using plasmids containing the ubiquitin C or elongation factor 1alpha promoter. Gene Ther , 8(20), 1539-46.

[17] Greenland, J. R., Geiben, R., Ghosh, S., Pastor, W. A., & Letvin, N. L. (2007). Plasmid DNA vaccine-elicited cellular immune responses limit in vivo vaccine antigen expression through Fas-mediated apoptosis. J Immunol , 178(9), 5652-8.

[18] Herweijer, H., Zhang, G., Subbotin, V. M., Budker, V., Williams, P., & Wolff, J. A. (2001). Time course of gene expression after plasmid DNA gene transfer to the liver. J Gene Med , 3(3), 280-91.

[19] Jaenisch, R., Schnieke, A., & Harbers, K. (1985). Treatment of mice with 5-azacytidine efficiently activates silent retroviral genomes in different tissues. Proc Natl Acad Sci U S A , 82(5), 1451-5.

[20] Jooss, K., Ertl, H. C., & Wilson, J. M. (1998). Cytotoxic T-lymphocyte target proteins and their major histocompatibility complex class I restriction in response to adenovirus vectors delivered to mouse liver. J Virol , 72(4), 2945-54.

[21] Jooss, K., Yang, Y., Fisher, K. J., & Wilson, J. M. (1998). Transduction of dendritic cells by DNA viral vectors directs the immune response to transgene products in muscle fibers. J Virol , 72(5), 4212-23.

[22] Kanai, Y. (2008). Alterations of DNA methylation and clinicopathological diversity of human cancers. Pathol Int , 58(9), 544-58.

[23] Louboutin, J. P., Wang, L., & Wilson, J. M. (2005). Gene transfer into skeletal muscle using novel AAV serotypes. J Gene Med , 7(4), 442-51.

[24] Mir, L. M., Bureau, M. F., Gehl, J., Rangara, R., Rouy, D., Caillaud, J. M., Delaere, P., Branellec, D., Schwartz, B., & Scherman, D. (1999). High-efficiency gene transfer into skeletal muscle mediated by electric pulses. Proc Natl Acad Sci U S A , 96(8), 4262-7.

[25] Momparler, R. L., & Bovenzi, V. (2000). DNA methylation and cancer. J Cell Physiol , 183(2), 145-54.

[26] Morrissey, D., van Pijkeren, J. P., Rajendran, S., Collins, S. A., Casey, G., O'Sullivan, G. C., & Tangney, M. (2012). Control and augmentation of long-term plasmid transgene expression in vivo in murine muscle tissue and ex vivo in patient mesenchymal tissue. J Biomed Biotechnol 2012: 3798451110-7251 (Electronic)1110-7243 (Linking)

[27] Ohlfest, J. R., Demorest, Z. L., Motooka, Y., Vengco, I., Oh, S., Chen, E., Scappaticci, F. A., Saplis, R. J., Ekker, S. C., Low, W. C., Freese, A. B., & Largaespada, D. A. (2005). Combinatorial antiangiogenic gene therapy by nonviral gene transfer using the sleeping beauty transposon causes tumor regression and improves survival in mice bearing intracranial human glioblastoma. Mol Ther , 12(5), 778-88.

[28]  Prosch, S., Stein, J., Staak, K., Liebenthal, C., Volk, H. D., & Kruger, D. H. (1996). Inactivation of the very strong HCMV immediate early promoter by DNA CpG methylation in vitro. Biol Chem Hoppe Seyler , 377(3), 195-201.

[29]  Sandrin, V., Russell, S. J., & Cosset, F. L. (2003). Targeting retroviral and lentiviral vectors." Curr Top Microbiol Immunol , 281, 137-78.

[30]  Scheule, R. K. (2000). The role of CpG motifs in immunostimulation and gene therapy. Adv Drug Deliv Rev 44(2-3): , 119 EOF-34 EOF.

[31]  Tang, Q., & Maul, G. G. (2003). Mouse cytomegalovirus immediate-early protein 1 binds with host cell repressors to relieve suppressive effects on viral transcription and replication during lytic infection. J Virol , 77(2), 1357-67.

[32]  Tangney, M., & Francis, K. P. (2012). In vivo optical imaging in gene & cell therapy." Curr Gene Ther 12(1): 2-111875-5631 (Electronic)1566-5232 (Linking)

[33]  Vanniasinkam, T., Ertl, H., & Tang, Q. (2006). Trichostatin-A enhances adaptive immune responses to DNA vaccination. J Clin Virol , 36(4), 292-7.

[34]  Wang, L., Dobrzynski, E., Schlachterman, A., Cao, O., & Herzog, R. W. (2005). Systemic protein delivery by muscle-gene transfer is limited by a local immune response. Blood, 105(11), 4226-34.

[35]  Yew, N. S., Przybylska, M., Ziegler, R. J., Liu, D., & Cheng, S. H. (2001). High and sustained transgene expression in vivo from plasmid vectors containing a hybrid ubiquitin promoter. Mol Ther , 4(1), 75-82.

[36]  Yuasa, K., Sakamoto, M., Miyagoe-Suzuki, Y., Tanouchi, A., Yamamoto, H., Li, J., Chamberlain, J. S., Xiao, X., & Takeda, S. (2002). Adeno-associated virus vector-mediated gene transfer into dystrophin-deficient skeletal muscles evokes enhanced immune response against the transgene product. Gene Ther , 9(23), 1576-88.

# Gene Therapy Tools: Synthetic

# Chapter 4

# DNA Electrotransfer: An Effective Tool for Gene Therapy

Aurore Burgain-Chain and Daniel Scherman

Additional information is available at the end of the chapter

## 1. Introduction

The concept of gene therapy was first introduced in the mid-80s, and is based on the delivery of genetic material (DNA or RNA) in the nucleus of patient cells, so that it is expressed and produces a therapeutic effect.

Different approaches can be considered:

- Correcting defective function by supplying a functional gene to the cells, thereby directly addressing the cause of a genetic disease.

- Transferring a gene encoding a therapeutic protein, in order to treat, prevent or slow the progression of certain diseases.

- Introducing a gene leading to the death of a diseased cell

- Introducing antisense DNA inhibiting the formation of a protein or the replication of a virus

Originally developed for monogenic diseases, and therefore associated with the compensation of genes whose alteration is responsible for diseases, the concept of gene therapy has rapidly expanded to the use of DNA as a new type of drug. Therefore, gene therapy leads to indications which are far beyond the case of genetic diseases, since a DNA drug can, in principle, replace any medication which will control protein synthesis. Gene therapy seems an alternative choice to fight against diseases currently treated imperfectly, or not treated with conventional pharmaceutical approaches.

In addition, gene therapy has many advantages compared to the administration of recombinant proteins. Indeed, recombinant proteins are costly and their elimination from the blood flow is fast, while gene therapy leads to a long-term and potentially regulated production of a therapeutic protein. Gene therapy also allows the localized expression of the transgene, avoiding any risk associated with the presence of a systemic exogenous protein.

The main limitation of current gene therapy is the development of effective gene transfer. Indeed, in order to reach the cell nucleus, the therapeutic gene has to cross several biological barriers. Therefore, the success of any gene therapy requires the development of efficient and appropriate methods and vectors for introducing the gene of interest into target cells. The ideal vehicle for gene transfer must have the following properties: (1) specificity to target cells, (2) localized gene delivery, (3) resistance to metabolic degradation and/or attack by the immune system, (4) minimum side effects, and (5) eventually controlled temporal transgene expression [1].

Many methods of *in vivo* gene transfer exist and are generally classified into two main categories: viral and non viral. Viruses are very efficient vehicles for gene transfer; however their use is limited by high production costs and safety concerns, such as immune response, possible pathogen reversion, mutagenesis and carcinogenesis. Considering these limitations, the delivery of therapeutic genes to target cells by non viral approaches may be of great value for the development of gene therapy. Among these approaches, *in vivo* electroporation, also called *in vivo* electropermeabilization or *in vivo* electrotransfer, has proven to be one of the simplest and most efficient methods for gene therapy, while at the same time being safe, cheap, and easy to perform.

*In vivo* electrotransfer is a recent physical technique for gene delivery in various tissues and organs, which relies on the combination of plasmid injection and delivery of short and defined electric pulses. This process results in the association between cell permeabilization and DNA electrophoresis. Skeletal muscle have now been frequently electrotransfered, since it offers promising treatment for muscle disorders, but also a way for systemic secretion of therapeutic proteins, by converting skeletal muscles into an endocrine organ: the protein produced can diffuse into the vascular system and circulate throughout the body to exert a physiological and potentially therapeutic effect. Many published studies have demonstrated that plasmid electrotransfer can lead to long-lasting therapeutic effects in various pathologies such as cancer, rheumatoid arthritis, muscle and blood disorders, cardiac diseases, etc... Indeed, the physical method of electrotransfer allows for greater efficiency of gene transfer after a single injection and improves protein expression by several orders of magnitude, as compared to DNA injected in the absence of electrotransfer. Therefore, plasmid electrotransfer can be considered a powerful tool for gene therapy.

The scope of this chapter encompasses the methods of electrotransfer, its implementation, mechanism, optimization and therapeutic applications.

## 2. Description of the electrotransfer technique

In 1982, E. Neumann and his collaborators demonstrated *in vitro* the possibility of introducing DNA into cells using electrical pulses [2]. These electric pulses would cause the destabilization and permeabilization of the plasma membrane of suspended cells, thus promoting the entry of exogenous DNA into these cells. Two years later [3], the confirmation of this result opened the way for the development of electroporation (or electropermeabilization) into bacterial [4], fungal [5] vegetal or animal cells. This method is routinely used now. The optimization of electrical parameters is critical to allow transient permeabilization, together with a satisfactory cell survival rate [6].

In initial studies, *in vivo* DNA electrotransfer has been tested in the skin in 1991, by the use of exponentially decaying electrical pulses, and in 1996 in the liver using trains of short 100 μs pulses [7]. In 1998, four independent teams showed the effectiveness of electrotransfer using pulses of long duration (5-50ms): in skeletal muscle, our team in collaboration with that of Luis Mir [8] and Aihara [9], in tumors, Rols *et al.* [10] and in liver Suzuki *et al.* [11]. *In vivo* DNA electrotransfer has now been successfully used in a broad range of target tissues and organs including for example : arteries [12], skin [13], tendon [14], bladder [15], cornea [16], the retinal cells [17], spinal cord [18]and brain [19].

Electropermeabilization can also be used to deliver chemical drugs into the cells: e.g. electro-chemotherapy in tumors, with the use of bleomycin, developed since 1991 [20]. Several clinical trials are underway [21], primarily for the treatment of subcutaneous or skin tumors [22, 23] and recently for the treatment of breast cancer with cisplatin [24] (For a review see [25]).

# 3. Mechanism of electrotransfer at the cell level

The technique of electroporation for the transfer of nucleic acids has been used since the 80s, however its exact mechanism is not yet completely elucidated [26, 27]. At the cell level, it seems that two phenomena occur: first the permeabilization of the cell to small molecules, probably due to a destabilization of the cell membrane, and secondly the transport of DNA by electrophoresis.

## 3.1. Permeabilization

The lipid bi-layer of the plasma membrane separates two solutions with very high ionic conductivity: the cytoplasm and the extracellular medium. Typically, at rest, the membrane potential difference ($\Delta Vm_0$) is around -70mV. When an electric field is applied to a cell, the resulting current induces an accumulation of electric charges at the cell membrane which leads to a variation of thistransmembrane potential. And if the transmembrane potential exceeds a certain threshold value, the cell membrane is disorganized and structural changes occur. That is a necessary condition for an effective gene transfer [28].

Shall the cell be considered a hollow sphere where the thickness of the membrane is negligible vis-à-vis the cell radius, then the transmembrane potential difference $\Delta Vm$ induced by an electric field is, as described by Schwann's equation:

$$\Delta Vm = f.g.r.E.cosq.(1-exp(-t/t)) \tag{1}$$

Thus, the transmembrane potential difference $\Delta Vm$ is proportional to

- the cell radius (r)
- the magnitude of the electric field (E) (expressed in volts/cm)
- the cosine of ($\theta$), its incidence angle,
- a cell shape factor (f)
- the conductivity of the medium (g)
- the pulse duration for which the electric field is applied (t)
- the charging time constant of the cell ($\tau$).

If the membrane is seen as a pure dielectric object, g is equal to 1. Under the conditions used for cellular electroporation, the pulse duration is significantly longer (of a few hundred microseconds to a few milliseconds) than the charging time constant of the cell, which is of the order of a few microseconds. The equation can be simplified to:

$$\Delta Vm = f. r.E.cosq \tag{2}$$

This transmembrane potential difference $\Delta Vm$ is not uniform on the surface of the cell: the induced transmembrane potential is maximal at the points of the cell facing the electrodes ($\theta = 0$ and $\pi$).

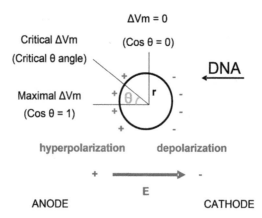

**Figure 1.** Theoretical model of the cell for electroporation: E, the electrical potential induces $\Delta Vm$, a transmembrane potential difference which dependent on r, the radius of the cell and $\theta$, the angle between the direction of electric field and the normal to the tangent of the membrane of the cell at this point

The membrane is off-balance and becomes transiently permeable when the sum: $\Delta Vm_0$ (at rest) + $\Delta Vm$ (induced) reaches a threshold value of about 200mV [29]. Thus, the greater the difference between the threshold value and the value applied, the greater the surface area is permeabilized. However for a given electric field, beyond a certain angle, the $\Delta Vm$ falls below the threshold value of permeabilization. The relationship between the applied electric field and the permeabilized surface was demonstrated by *in vitro* fluorescent labeling of permeabilized areas of the cell [30]. Moreover, these studies have shown that it is the face of the cell toward the anode side which is permeabilized first, the negative potential of the cell being in addition to that induced by the external electric field.

One theory suggests that the DNA enters into the cell through pores which are generated by electrical stimulation [32]. The electropermeabilization creates relatively stable "electropores" [2, 33]. But these pores have never been visualized. The plasmid DNA may optionally pass the membrane after a step of binding to the surface of the cell and by diffusion.

The second phenomenon necessary for gene transfer by electroporation is the electrophoresis of negatively charged DNA.

### 3.2. DNA electrophoresis

The occurrence of an electrophoretic process has been demonstrated *in vitro* [31]. Various studies have shown this electrophoretic effect: Klenchin *et al.* demonstrated that DNA has to be present at the time of the pulses [31]. Furthermore, they showed that the transfection efficiency depends on the polarity of the electric field. Sukharev *et al.* also showed *in vitro* that short pulses of high voltage (HV) induce membrane permeabilization but not transfection, whereas long pulses at low voltage (LV) do not induce permeabilization or transfection. However, the sequence "high voltage pulses followed by low voltage pulses" provides a transfection. An hypothesis is proposed that transfection of cells permeabilized by high voltage is only possible if low voltage pulses can subsequently mediate DNA electrophoresis [34].

The role of permeabilization and electrophoresis was demonstrated directly at the cell level by fluorescence microscopy [35]. This work shows that interaction between the membrane and electropermeabilized DNA is induced in response to electrical pulses of a few milliseconds. DNA electrophoretically accumulates on the cathode side of the cell without immediately moving into the cytosol (Figure 1). Thus DNA must be present during the pulse and electrophoresis induced by the electric field promotes its transfer through the membrane, but it is only during the following minute that DNA crosses the electropermeabilized membrane [36]. There is a direct relationship between the DNA/membrane interaction and transfection efficiency: the larger the contact surface between DNA and the membrane, the higher is the expression [27].

## 4. Mechanism of *in vivo* electrotransfer

In the early 90's, the first studies about *in vivo* electroporation appeared. They primarily concerned the transfer of chemical molecules. The first real demonstration of *in vivo* cellular electropermeabilization was performed on tumors after injection of bleomycin, a cytotoxic anticancer agent, [22, 37]. The effectiveness of bleomycin depends on its intracellular concentration, but this drug penetrates poorly into cells. Therefore, a better penetration of bleomycin was measured after application of electric pulses to tumors, leading to an enhanced desired cytotoxicity.

Most studies are pointing to a mechanism of *in vivo* electrotransfer comparable to the mechanism of *in vitro* electrotransfer described above,which can be extended to the whole tissue: several steps have to take place, including cell permeabilization beyond a threshold value of local electric field. In 1999, we evaluated on one hand cell permeabilization following the application of electrical pulses by measuring the ability of muscle cells to capture a small radioactive hydrophilic molecule complexe of EDTA Chelating 51 chromium ($^{51}$Cr-EDTA), and on the other hand, transgene expression for evidence of DNA entry [38, 39]. The uptake of $^{51}$Cr-EDTA was similar whether injected thirty seconds before or after applying electrical pulses. In contrast, DNA injected after the electrical impulses does not penetrate into cells. This suggests that DNA must be present *in situ* at the time of electrical pulses to obtain an efficient cell transfection, and that there is a direct, active effect of the electric field on the DNA molecules to promote their entry into cells. Hence the current mechanistic hypothesis of gene electrotransfer necessitates not only a permeabilization of cell membranes but also a DNA electrophoresis.

This hypothesis is supported by the study of Bureau *et al.* [40] of gene electrotransfer in skeletal muscle of mice with different combinations of long pulses of low voltage (LV, i.e. electrophoretic pulses) and short pulses of high voltage (HV, i.e. permeabilizing pulses). Only the combination of a HV-pulse followed by a LV-pulse provided efficient gene transfer. Further studies confirmed that HV-pulses are related to permeabilization, while LV-pulses are related to the efficiency of DNA electrophoresis [41]. The importance of cell permeabilization was also studied by magnetic resonance imaging using a gadolinium complex as contrast agent (dimeglumine gadopentate): the zone of di meglumine gadopentate complex permeabilization is identical to the area expression of electrotransfered DNA [42].

The destabilization of cell membranes and the electrophoretic effect are probably not the only mechanisms involved in gene transfer by electroporation. Scientists have discussed the importance of energy metabolism (ATP and ADP) for the passage of DNA through the permeabilized membrane and its migration to the nucleus [28].

Other studies suggest a mechanism of DNA transport by endocytosis [43]. These same studies show that transfection efficiency does not decrease if the electrical pulses are delivered up to four hours after injection of DNA, while other studies show that most of the injected DNA is degraded in first hours after injection [44]. We also confirmed that after an intramuscular injection, most of the DNA is degraded and eliminated quickly. However, a small proportion of DNA is preserved and provides a source of stable DNA which can been electrotransfered [45].

In summary, the molecular mechanism of *in vivo* DNA electrotransfer is still under investigation. It likely corresponds to multiple steps whose elucidation and understanding of respective contribution could help to develop more effective electrotransfer strategies and protocols.

## 5. Electrotransfer into practice

The *in vivo* electrotransfer technique is particularly easy to implement: a solution of plasmid DNA (i. e. a circular nucleic acid) in isotonic saline (NaCl, 150mM) is injected into the target tissue with a syringe, and electric pulses are then delivered by means of electrodes placed on either side of the injection site and connected to a generator (Figure 2). Electrodes can be either needles or plates.

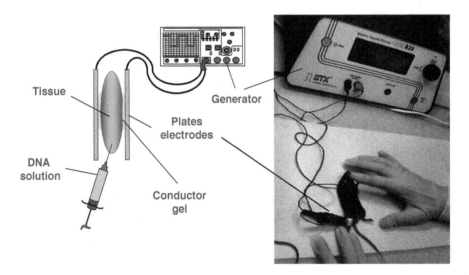

**Figure 2.** Experimental set up for intramuscular plasmid electrotransfer in mice

This technique allows a site specific gene transfer. It is relatively efficient in skeletal muscle and is applicable to many other tissues such as brain, liver, skin, bladder, kidney, lung, cornea, retina, testis, tumor tissue etc... for more details see [46]. Electrotransfer can also be used in a wealth of animal models, ranging from rats and mice to sheeps [47] and cows [48] and even fish [49].

### 5.1. Operating parameters

The efficiency of gene transfer depends on the target tissue, the delivered DNA and electric pulses parameters. The aim is to deliver, into each tissue, electrical pulses that can cause the permeabilization of cell membranes and DNA transfer, while remaining below the toxic threshold. Otherwise, local cell death by necrosis of the treated cells would occur, followe by tissue regeneration, which would induce the loss of the benefit of the treatment (but with no toxicity at the level of the whole organism). Therefore, optimal conditions for the DNA electrotransfer in a targeted tissue result from a compromise between the efficiency of DNA transfer and minimal cellular toxicity.

### 5.1.1. The electrodes

The choice of electrodes depends on the target tissue and the size of the treated animal. It is critically important and should be carefully considered. For an electrotransfer on a small animal in a tissue such as skeletal muscle, or liver tumor, most experimenters use electrodes made of two plates attached to a clamp (Figure 3, left). Indeed, this type of electrodes can be easily applied externally on each side of the interested tissue. Because one key parameter is the electric field, which is related to the ratio between the voltage applied and the distance between electrodes, this latter distance should not be too large in order to avoid prohibitive high voltage *in vivo* delivery. Thus, for animals of larger size, needle electrodes (Figure 3, right) are more often used than external plates.

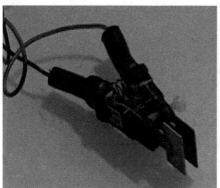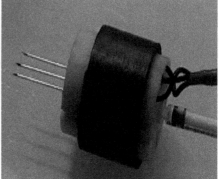

**Figure 3.** Examples of electrode plates for external use (left) and needle electrodes for internal use, designed by the company Sphergen (right).

### 5.1.2. Electrical parameters

Knowing the magnitude and distribution of electric field is very important for both efficient gene transfer and reduced toxicity. The distribution of the electric field is dependent on both the tissue and the type of electrodes, which causes variations in the effective magnitude of the field in the tissue area of interest. The electric field distribution is more homogeneous when using plate electrodes than with needle electrodes, and for a given setting, the resulting electric field is lower with needle electrodes that with electrode plates [38].

Moreover, it is necessary to determine, for each tissue and each species, the threshold values of the electric field magnitude, i.e. the permeabilization threshold (reversible) and the cell damage threshold (irreversible), in order to define optimal electrical conditions for gene transfer with minimal toxic effects. Micklavic *et al.* have developed a system combining numerical predictions and experimental observations in order to determine these thresholds in the case of needle electrodes used in rat liver for drug delivery [50].

Different types of electrical pulses can be applied: unipolar square pulses, bipolar square pulses, or pulses with exponential decay [51]. The exponentially decaying pulses, colloquially referred to as "exponential pulses" are mainly used *in vitro* with a time constant dependent on the resistance of the incubation media. The square pulses are preferred *in vivo*, since the voltage and pulse duration can be set independently of the electrical resistance of the targeted tissue. Unipolar square pulses are the most widely used for electrotransfer experiments, while bipolar squares pulses are rather used for electrophysiology [52].

## 5.2. Toxicity

Tissue damage can be caused by electrotransfer and thus limits the efficiency of transfection [53]. The cell permeabilization is the main toxicity factor: it leads to an inward diffusion of the external medium as well as leakage of intracellular content, thus changing the composition of the latter. This toxicity can be reduced by minimizing the duration and the extent of permeabilization.

Other factors of toxicity have been described such as oxidative stress due to the formation of free radicals near the electropermeabilized membrane [6, 54]. It was also shown that electrotransfer induced muscle damage dependent on the amount of DNA injected [55]; these lesions disappear within two months after injection.

In our laboratory, histological analyzes of muscle slices have shown that the application of electric fields optimized for gene transfer does not induce gene expression markers of stress and cellular toxicity [56]. Other experiments have allowed to conclude that, even in optimized conditions, very little muscle damage is generated: few inflammatory lesions are observed with a maximum in the first seven days after the electrotransfer, but these disappear rapidly in less than three weeks [57-58].

It is also possible to reduce the extent of damage by increasing the accessibility of DNA to target cells. Indeed, studies have shown that improving the plasmid distribution leads to an increase in transgene expression. Thus, the value of the electric field used can be reduced. Better distribution can be obtained for example by pre-injection of hyaluronidase [59], an enzyme that degrades hyaluronic acid, which is a major component of the extracellular matrix [60]. This pretreatment allows for the same expression level, using lower voltages while reducing muscle damage [61]. A pre-injection of sucrose may also improve the distribution of DNA, by creating spaces between the muscle fibers [62]. Similarly, a pre-injection of poly-L-glutamate, an anionic polymer, seems to increase the internalization of the plasmid inside the cell and/or to reduce its degradation [63], and therefore increases the expression of exogenous gene

## 5.3. Target tissues

During recent years, electrotransfer has been applied in various animal species to many tissues, including skeletal muscle, skin, liver, lungs, kidneys, joints, brain, retina, cornea, etc... [64]. The optimal parameters of a given electrotransfer should be determined based on the cell type and species, since these parameters strongly depend on tissue organization and the size of the transfected cells.

### 5.3.1. Skeletal muscle

One of the most widely used tissues for electrotransfer is skeletal muscle. The DNA electrotransfer into skeletal muscle was discovered independently by three teams [8, 9, 52]. Indeed, skeletal muscle offers many advantages:

- a large, easy access;
- sets of muscle fibers are parallel to each other: many fibers might have an optimal orientation relative to the electric field, which promotes even transfer across the entire length of the fibers;
- unlike other cells, muscle cells have multiple nuclei flattened against the cell membrane, which facilitates DNA trafficking to the nucleus;
- muscle fibers do not divide, ensuring long-term gene expression, notwithstanding the absence of regeneration due to injury or cytotoxic immune response;
- finally, a major advantage of skeletal muscle lies in its ability to produce and release biologically active proteins into the bloodstream, due to the strong vascularisation.

Combined together, these features can turn muscle into systemic drug delivery system for distant targets [65]. Interestingly, the cotransfection of multiple unlinked genes can be easily performed by electroporation [66]. For examples of electrotransfer in skeletal muscle in various mammalian species see [46].

### 5.3.2. The skin

The skin is, as muscle, also a widely used tissue for DNA electrotransfer, mostly because:

- this tissue is easily accessible and a large area of tissue can be treated;
- keratinocytes, which are epidermal cells, can synthesize and secrete therapeutic proteins that reach the bloodstream;
- by its natural function of a biological barrier, the skin contains cells that present antigens and is therefore an organ of choice for applications in DNA vaccination;
- the epidermal cells have a short lifespan, which can be useful for treatments requiring a brief period of expression.

However, skin structure [67] does not facilitate gene transfer. In particular, the top layer (stratum corneum or horny layer) is a major barrier [68, 69]. But a high level of expression in the skin from a single injection could still be observed [70, 71]. Moreover Dujardin *et al.* have shown that square or exponential pulses induce moderate and reversible effects on the skin without inflammation or necrosis, while transiently permeabilizing the skin and thus allowing the passage of molecules [72].

### 5.4. Optimization of *in vivo* electrotransfer conditions

An important goal for gene transfer applications is the level and duration of gene expression. To determine optimal conditions which maximize efficiency while reducing tissue damage, different protocols have been used to improve the access of plasmids to targeted cells. As already described, improved plasmid distribution in the skeletal muscle leads to an increase in DNA expression. Accordingly, Cemazar *et al.* showed recently enhanced transfection efficiency of gene transfer by pretreatment of tumors with hyaluronidase and/or collagenase, two enzymes which modulate components of the extracellular matrix [73].

A secretion signal can be also added to the transgene sequence : we have recently shown that by modifying the cellular localization of the produced protein by adding a secretory signal, the production and secretion of this protein is enhanced, thus enhancing biological effect [74].

We have also shown that codon optimization of the transgene (i.e. retaining the natural amino acid sequence but using the preferred host animal codons) leads to increase in the expression of the protein of interest [74].

Another method to increase the stability of the protein produced in the blood circulation is to increase its size in order to avoid kidney excretion. Thus, the construction of fusion proteins, for instance by fusing a therapeutic protein with an IgG constant [75], appears a simple way to deliver enhanced levels of secreted proteins without altering their biological activities.

The enhanced protein expression, and so their biological effects, also depends of the injection regimen and the administered plasmid dose [74].

## 6. Applications of plasmid electrotransfer

DNA electrotransfer is a recent technique of has not yet successfully completed all stages of clinical development, but this is progressing. The first Phase I human clinical trial has been initiated in U.S. by the company Inovio Biomedicals, for the treatment of skin cancer [76]. Since then, the delivery of plasmid DNA encoding therapeutic genes has been tested extensively in preclinical melanoma models [77].

Applications designated as "therapeutic" which are mainly reported in the literature have been demonstrated on animal models of human diseases. The main potential therapeutic areas cover cancer [78], cardiovascular diseases [75], autoimmune diseases [79], monogenic diseases [80], organ-specific disorders [81] and vaccination [82, 83]. Different examples show

the efficiency of plasmid electrotransfer to produce therapeutic proteins in various pathologies [46]: all these experiments showed an improvement in symptoms of the relative disorder.

## 6.1. Cancer

Cancer accounts for major field of application trials of gene therapy. Different strategies can
be broadly grouped into four main categories:

a.   Stimulation of the immune response against a tumor [84],

b.   Use of suicide genes [85-87];

c.   Repair cell cycle defects caused by the loss of tumor suppressor genes or oncogene acti-
     vation [88],

d.   Inhibition of tumor angiogenesis [89].

These strategies can be combined to obtain synergistic results. For example, a combination
of HSV-TK-suicide gene therapy and IL-21 immune gene therapy byelectrotransfer improves antitumor responses in mice [90]. Moreover, *in vivo* electrotransfer could be used in
combination with other strategies such as chemotherapy, because these two approaches use
different mechanisms to kill cancer cells, and thus a synergistic effect may be obtained.

Actually, electroporation of DNA encoding cytokines into tumors is extensively studied:
IL-12 [91], IL-18 [92], IFN-$\alpha$ [93] have been shown to reduce tumor growth and increase survival times in different tumor models. Other interesting results are represented by the inhibition of tumor growth in various models with plasmids encoding metaloproteinase-3
inhibitor for the treatment of prostate cancers [94], or encoding endostatin for his therapeutic efficacy in mouse-transplanted tumors [95].

All these experiments show the potential of in vivo electrotranfer for cancer treatment.
And the strategy used, i.e. the direct intra-tumoral plasmid electrotransfer, is well suited
for the local production of therapeutic proteins. However, since the efficacy of gene
transfer into tumor cells *in vivo* is generally low, intramuscular electrotransfer can also
be efficiently used for distal tumor treatment. Indeed, an important application of the
technique of plasmid electrotransfer is the protein secretion by skeletal muscle: the produced protein, such as, for instant, an immunostimulating cytokine, can diffuse into the
vascular system and circulate throughout the body to exert a physiological effect, particularly therapeutic. This distal approach may be very powerful for surgically inaccessible
tumors, such as head and neck tumors.

Finally, the intramuscular electrotransfer of a plasmid encoding the prostate membrane specific antigen (PMSA) has been tested in a human clinical trial of prostate cancer active immunotherapy [96]. DNA fusion-gene vaccination in patients with prostate cancer induces
high-frequency CD8 (+) T-cell responses and increases PSA doubling time [97].

## 6.2. Monogenic diseases

Monogenic diseases with an identified defective gene have been the first diseases targeted by gene therapy approaches. Among these diseases, Duchenne muscular dystrophy (DMD), which is characterized by the absence of dystrophin, is a good model, since even a small amount of dystrophin would be sufficient to reverse the clinical phenotype of the disease. An approach to eventually restore this protein in patients with DMD is to introduce into their muscles a plasmid encoding dystrophinc DNA. Pichavant *et al.* were the first to demonstrate local restoration of full-length dog dystrophin in dystrophic dog muscle by DNA electrotransfer [98].

## 6.3. Hematopoietic factor deficiency

Erythropoietin (EPO) is another good candidate for gene therapy applications because a small amount will produce the desired physiological effect of raising the hematocrit. Numerous studies, in particular by our own group, report efficient EPO secretion after plasmid electrotransfer, with a therapeutic effect in anemia and beta thalassemia. The use of intramuscular plasmid electrotransfer for EPO gene delivery in mice increased approximately 10 to 100-fold the expression of this gene, as compared to naked DNA alone [99, 100]. Moreover with this method, the protein in circulation and hematocrit levels were stable for 2 to 6 months after a single injection of minimal amounts (as little as 1 μg) of a plasmid carrying the mouse EPO cDNA. Several studies also showed that EPO expression could be regulated, for instance by co-administering an EPO encoding plasmid under the control of a tetracycline-inducible promotor and a second plasmid carrying the reverse tetracycline-dependent transactivator protein [100, 101]. All these studies exemplified that plasmid DNA electrotransfer can efficiently produce enough amounts of transgenic EPO in normal mice.

In collaboration with the group of Y. Beuzard, we have demonstrated the relevance of intramuscular electroporation of an EPO-expressing plasmid in a mouse model of human β-thalassemia, a severe genetic disease, leading to a durable and dose-dependent phenotypic correction of this severe genetic disease [102]. In addition, we have also shown that it is possible to produce fusion protein by plasmid DNA electrotransfer [103]: indeed since the bridging of two adjacent EPO receptors triggers a conformational change that initiates signal transduction [104], we have hypothesized that the fusion of two EPO molecules might lead an increase in intrinsic activity of EPO. Thus, we demonstrated that the injection of EPO dimer encoding plasmid by electrotransfer in a skeletal muscle of β-thalassemic mice induces an increase in the biologic specific activity of this EPO dimer in comparison with the activity of monomer [103].

Furthermore the secretion peak of therapeutic protein following DNA administration is potentially deleterious. We reported that muscular electrotransfer of low doses of plasmid can be repeated several times to weeks or even months after the initial injection, and that this strategy leads to efficient, long-lasting and non-toxic treatment of β-thalassemic mouse anemia avoiding the deleterious initial hematocrit peak and maintaining a normal hematocrit with small fluctuation [105].

In addition, Gothelf *et al.* demonstrate that gene electrotransfer to skin of even small amounts of EPO DNA can lead to systemically therapeutic levels of EPO protein [106].

## 6.4. Cardiovascular diseases

Gene therapy is an attractive strategy for the treatment of cardiovascular disease. However, using current methods, the induction of gene expression at therapeutic levels is often inefficient. Therefore DNA electrotransfer directly into heart may enhance the delivery of therapeutic protein as shown the team of R. Heller : the electroporation method ameliorates the delivery of a plasmid encoding an angiogenic growth factor (vascular endothelial growth factor, VEGF), which is a molecule previously documented to stimulate revascularization in coronary artery disease [107]. Ayuni *et al.* demonstrated that, unlike the usual methods to treat coronary artery diseases, electrotransfer applied directly into the beating heart enhances the delivery of a plasmid injected via the coronary veins after transient occlusion of the coronary sinus [108]. These results show that *in vivo* electroporation mediated gene transfer is feasible and safe,in particular to the heart. Finally, in skin, D. Dean reported that using electroporation in skin enhances delivery of plasmid DNA encoding fibroblast growth factor-2 (FGF-2) to induce neovascularization as atherapy for ischemia in a rat model [109].

## 6.5. Eye diseases

The eye is an isolated organ difficult to reach via systemic administration. Eye diseases are treated with intra- or periocular injections and these repeated injections bear the risk of adverse effects, mainly infections, and are poorly tolerated by the patients. The use of DNA electrotransfer technique is therefore possible to deliver a local treatment. Our team associated with an ophtalmology group has developed electrotransfer to the ciliary muscle, which is a particular smooth muscle with some characteristics of striated skeletal muscle, for the local treatment of inflammatory eye disease. This approach led to production and secretion of therapeutic levels of TNFα soluble receptor in the ocular media, and not in the serum, thus preventing clinical and histological signs in a rat uveitis model [110, 111]. Recently, suprachoroidal electrotransfer with a reporter plasmid to transfect the choroid and the retina without detaching the retina has been reported [112]. Not only choroidal cells but also RPE, and potentially photoreceptors, were efficiently transduced for at least a month, without ocular complications. This minimally invasive non-viral gene therapy method may open new prospects for human retinal therapies.

## 6.6. Obesity and diabetes

As mentioned above, skeletal muscle can be an efficient platform for the secretion of erythropoietin (EPO), which displays a variety of metabolic effects when it is expressed in supraphysiological levels. Hojman *et al.* have proposed to overexpress EPO in muscle by electrotransfer of plasmid in the aim to protect mice against diet-induced obesity and normalize glucose sensitivity, associated with a shift to increased fat metabolism in the muscles [113]. Similar results were obtained after DNA electrotransfer of plasmid encoding the carnitine palmitoyltransferase 1 (CPT1), the enzyme that controls the entry of long-chain fatty ac-yl CoA into mitochondria: an overexpression of CPT1 led to enhance rates of fatty acid beta-oxidation and improved insulin action in muscle in high-fat diet insulin-resistant rats [114]. In the same model, electrotransfer of the orphan nuclear receptor (Nur77) significantly amel-iorates the effect of this protein on glucose metabolism [115].

### 6.7. Vaccination and passive immunization by antibody production

The prospect of inducing an immune response to a protein expressed *in vivo* directly from administered DNA vaccine represents an attractive alternative to other modes of vaccina-tion. Plasmid electrotransfer has been used in genetic immunization to produce antigenic proteins. It is now well established that genetic immunization induces both durable cellular and humoral responses [116]. This type of immunization is often developed for vaccination (virus or antibacterial), for anticancer active immunotherapy, and also to induce in animals the production with high yield of antibodies against a given antigen.

Since electrotransfer efficiently transfers genes compared to a single injection of plasmid, improving antigenic protein expression by several orders of magnitude, the antibody tit-er and the quality of the immune response are also improved [117], with an increasing factor of 100 in mice after electrotransfer of a plasmid encoding a surface antigen of hep-atitis B [118]. High titers of antibodies were also obtained in mice and rabbits after i.m. electrotransfer of a plasmid encoding an envelope glycoprotein of hepatitis C [119], and in mice after electrotransfer of a plasmid encoding a protein of Mycobacterium tubercu-losis [120]. In the laboratory, it was shown that i.m. electrotransfer of a plasmid encod-ing the influenza hemagglutinin induces a better immune response in mice that a single i.m. injection [121]. And recently, we have assessed the potential of i.m. electrotransferin mouse to produce neutralizing antibodies, with high titer, against botulinum toxins, the most powerful poison in the world in present time [74]. We have optimized DNA elec-trotransfer for genetic immunization against botulinum antigen. This DNA immunization has been used in rabbits to induce antibodies production which is compatible with in-dustrial development of antiserum production for a human therapeutic use (Burgain *et al.*, unpublished results).These examples show that it is possible to obtain high titers neu-tralizing antibodies in animals by DNA electrotransfer.

Monoclonal antibodies are increasingly being used in a wide range of clinical applications in the field of autoimmune disease, cancer and infectious disease. The production and secre-tion by electrotransfered muscle of monoclonal antibodies has been demonstrated by our group and the one of I. Mathiesen, independently [83, 122]. These studies demonstrated that the co-transfection of two naked plasmids encoding the heavy and light G immunoglobulin chains led to the secretion of fully assembled and functional immunoglobulin molecules. The successful neutralization of various pathogens resulted from monoclonal antibody se-cretion by electrotransfered muscle, raising the possibility of clinical passive immunization applications.

# 7. Conclusion

*In vivo* electrotransfer is a non-viral technique which has emerged as an efficient, user-friendly and cheap gene transfer method which issuited for a wide range of tissues and species. Moreover, *in vivo* electrotransfer can be used for either local or distal effect by secretion of the transgenic protein into the bloodstream. The skeletal muscle is able to produce functional proteins with adequate post-translational modifications, which means that the muscle can be used as an endocrine organ for the production of therapeutic secreted proteins targeting systemic diseases. It is now established that therapeutic levels of circulating proteins can be reached in animal models. And since DNA does not induce any immune response, plasmid electrotransfer can be repeated as often as desired (Scherman *et al.*, unpublished results).

The understanding of the precise mechanism of electrotransfer, the optimization of its realization, the improvement of plasmids and of the structure of the encoded protein will bring more efficiency and above all more safety to the method, should it be applied to humans. Several clinical trials have been conducted and/or are still in progress. For more details see http://www.clinicaltrials.gov/ct2/results?term=electroporation. These clinical trials are mainly conducted against infectious diseases such AIDS, hepatitis B, malaria, dengue, influenza... and various cancer types such as ovarian cancer or renal cancer, melanoma, cancers caused by human papillomavirus... Thus, DNA electrotransfer appears as a powerful and promising tool not only for gene therapy, but also for in vivo gene delivery at the laboratory level within the frame of physiological studies.

## Author details

Aurore Burgain-Chain and Daniel Scherman

Unit of Chemical and Genetic Pharmacology and of Bioimaging, CNRS Paris, Université Paris Descartes; Chimie Paris Tech; Paris-Sorbonne PRES, France

## References

[1]  Mehier-Humbert S, Guy RH. Physical methods for gene transfer: improving the kinetics of gene delivery into cells. Adv Drug Deliv Rev. 2005 Apr 5;57(5):733-53.

[2]  Neumann E, Schaefer-Ridder M, Wang Y, Hofschneider PH. Gene transfer into mouse lyoma cells by electroporation in high electric fields. Embo J. 1982;1(7):841-5.

[3]  Potter H, Weir L, Leder P. Enhancer-dependent expression of human kappa immunoglobulin genes introduced into mouse pre-B lymphocytes by electroporation. Proc NatlAcadSci U S A. 1984 Nov;81(22):7161-5.

[4] Calvin NM, Hanawalt PC. High-efficiency transformation of bacterial cells by electroporation. J Bacteriol. 1988 Jun;170(6):2796-801.

[5] Ganeva V, Galutzov B, Teissie J. Fast kinetic studies of plasmid DNA transfer in intact yeast cells mediated by electropulsation. BiochemBiophys Res Commun. 1995 Sep 25;214(3):825-32.

[6] Bonnafous P, Vernhes M, Teissie J, Gabriel B. The generation of reactive-oxygen species associated with long-lasting pulse-induced electropermeabilisation of mammalian cells is based on a non-destructive alteration of the plasma membrane. BiochimBiophysActa. 1999 Nov 9;1461(1):123-34.

[7] Heller R, Jaroszeski M, Atkin A, Moradpour D, Gilbert R, Wands J, et al. In vivo gene electroinjection and expression in rat liver. FEBS Lett. 1996 Jul 8;389(3):225-8.

[8] Mir LM, Bureau MF, Rangara R, Schwartz B, Scherman D. Long-term, high level in vivo gene expression after electric pulse-mediated gene transfer into skeletal muscle. C R AcadSci III. 1998 Nov;321(11):893-9.

[9] Aihara H, Miyazaki J. Gene transfer into muscle by electroporation in vivo. Nat Biotechnol. 1998 Sep;16(9):867-70.

[10] Rols MP, Delteil C, Golzio M, Dumond P, Cros S, Teissie J. In vivo electrically mediated protein and gene transfer in murine melanoma. Nat Biotechnol. 1998 Feb;16(2): 168-71.

[11] Suzuki T, Shin BC, Fujikura K, Matsuzaki T, Takata K. Direct gene transfer into rat liver cells by in vivo electroporation. FEBS Lett. 1998 Apr 3;425(3):436-40.

[12] Matsumoto T, Komori K, Shoji T, Kuma S, Kume M, Yamaoka T, et al. Successful and optimized in vivo gene transfer to rabbit carotid artery mediated by electronic pulse. Gene Ther. 2001 Aug;8(15):1174-9.

[13] Maruyama H, Ataka K, Higuchi N, Sakamoto F, Gejyo F, Miyazaki J. Skin-targeted gene transfer using in vivo electroporation. Gene Ther. 2001 Dec;8(23):1808-12.

[14] Jayankura M, Boggione C, Frisen C, Boyer O, Fouret P, Saillant G, et al. In situ gene transfer into animal tendons by injection of naked DNA and electrotransfer. J Gene Med. 2003 Jul;5(7):618-24.

[15] Harimoto K, Sugimura K, Lee CR, Kuratsukuri K, Kishimoto T. In vivo gene transfer methods in the bladder without viral vectors. Br J Urol. 1998 Jun;81(6):870-4.

[16] Blair-Parks K, Weston BC, Dean DA. High-level gene transfer to the cornea using electroporation. J Gene Med. 2002 Jan-Feb;4(1):92-100.

[17] Dezawa M, Takano M, Negishi H, Mo X, Oshitari T, Sawada H. Gene transfer into retinal ganglion cells by in vivo electroporation: a new approach. Micron. 2002;33(1): 1-6.

[18] Lin CR, Tai MH, Cheng JT, Chou AK, Wang JJ, Tan PH, et al. Electroporation for direct spinal gene transfer in rats. NeurosciLett. 2002 Jan 4;317(1):1-4.

[19] Inoue T, Krumlauf R. An impulse to the brain--using in vivo electroporation. Nat Neurosci. 2001 Nov;4 Suppl:1156-8.

[20] Mir LM, Belehradek M, Domenge C, Orlowski S, Poddevin B, Belehradek J, Jr., et al. [Electrochemotherapy, a new antitumor treatment: first clinical trial]. C R AcadSci III. 1991;313(13):613-8.

[21] Gothelf A, Mir LM, Gehl J. Electrochemotherapy: results of cancer treatment using enhanced delivery of bleomycin by electroporation. Cancer Treat Rev. 2003 Oct;29(5): 371-87.

[22] Mir LM, Glass LF, Sersa G, Teissie J, Domenge C, Miklavcic D, et al. Effective treatment of cutaneous and subcutaneous malignant tumours by electrochemotherapy. Br J Cancer. 1998 Jun;77(12):2336-42.

[23] Rols MP, Bachaud JM, Giraud P, Chevreau C, Roche H, Teissie J. Electrochemotherapy of cutaneous metastases in malignant melanoma. Melanoma Res. 2000 Oct;10(5): 468-74.

[24] Rebersek M, Cufer T, Cemazar M, Kranjc S, Sersa G. Electrochemotherapy with cisplatin of cutaneous tumor lesions in breast cancer. Anticancer Drugs. 2004 Jul;15(6): 593-7.

[25] Sersa G, Miklavcic D, Cemazar M, Rudolf Z, Pucihar G, Snoj M. Electrochemotherapy in treatment of tumours. Eur J SurgOncol. 2008 Feb;34(2):232-40.

[26] Escoffre JM, Portet T, Wasungu L, Teissie J, Dean D, Rols MP. What is (still not) known of the mechanism by which electroporation mediates gene transfer and expression in cells and tissues.MolBiotechnol. 2009 Mar;41(3):286-95.

[27] Faurie C, Phez E, Golzio M, Vossen C, Lesbordes JC, Delteil C, et al. Effect of electric field vectoriality on electrically mediated gene delivery in mammalian cells. BiochimBiophysActa. 2004 Oct 11;1665(1-2):92-100.

[28] Rols MP, Delteil C, Golzio M, Teissie J. Control by ATP and ADP of voltage-induced mammalian-cell-membrane permeabilization, gene transfer and resulting expression. Eur J Biochem. 1998 Jun 1;254(2):382-8.

[29] Teissie J, Rols MP. An experimental evaluation of the critical potential difference inducing cell membrane electropermeabilization. Biophys J. 1993 Jul;65(1):409-13.

[30] Gabriel B, Teissie J. Direct observation in the millisecond time range of fluorescent molecule asymmetrical interaction with the electropermeabilized cell membrane. Biophys J. 1997 Nov;73(5):2630-7.

[31] Klenchin VA, Sukharev SI, Serov SM, Chernomordik LV, Chizmadzhev Yu A. Electrically induced DNA uptake by cells is a fast process involving DNA electrophoresis. Biophys J. 1991 Oct;60(4):804-11.

[32] Xie TD, Sun L, Tsong TY. Study of mechanisms of electric field-induced DNA transfection. I. DNA entry by surface binding and diffusion through membrane pores. Biophys J. 1990 Jul;58(1):13-9.

[33] deGennes PG. Passive entry of a DNA molecule into a small pore. ProcNatlAcadSci U S A. 1999 Jun 22;96(13):7262-4.

[34] Sukharev SI, Klenchin VA, Serov SM, Chernomordik LV, Chizmadzhev Yu A. Electroporation and electrophoretic DNA transfer into cells. The effect of DNA interaction with electropores. Biophys J. 1992 Nov;63(5):1320-7.

[35] Golzio M, Teissie J, Rols MP. Direct visualization at the single-cell level of electrically mediated gene delivery. ProcNatlAcadSci U S A. 2002 Feb 5;99(3):1292-7.

[36] Golzio M, Rols MP, Teissie J. In vitro and in vivo electric field-mediated permeabilization, gene transfer, and expression. Methods. 2004 Jun;33(2):126-35.

[37] Belehradek J, Jr., Orlowski S, Ramirez LH, Pron G, Poddevin B, Mir LM. Electropermeabilization of cells in tissues assessed by the qualitative and quantitative electroloading of bleomycin. BiochimBiophysActa. 1994 Feb 23;1190(1):155-63.

[38] Gehl J, Sorensen TH, Nielsen K, Raskmark P, Nielsen SL, Skovsgaard T, et al. In vivo electroporation of skeletal muscle: threshold, efficacy and relation to electric field distribution. BiochimBiophysActa. 1999 Aug 5;1428(2-3):233-40.

[39] Mir LM, Bureau MF, Gehl J, Rangara R, Rouy D, Caillaud JM, et al. High-efficiency gene transfer into skeletal muscle mediated by electric pulses. ProcNatlAcadSci U S A. 1999 Apr 13;96(8):4262-7.

[40] Bureau MF, Gehl J, Deleuze V, Mir LM, Scherman D. Importance of association between permeabilization and electrophoretic forces for intramuscular DNA electrotransfer. BiochimBiophysActa. 2000 May 1;1474(3):353-9.

[41] Satkauskas S, Bureau MF, Puc M, Mahfoudi A, Scherman D, Miklavcic D, et al. Mechanisms of in vivo DNA electrotransfer: respective contributions of cell electropermeabilization and DNA electrophoresis. MolTher. 2002 Feb;5(2):133-40.

[42] Paturneau-Jouas M, Parzy E, Vidal G, Carlier PG, Wary C, Vilquin JT, et al. Electrotransfer at MR imaging: tool for optimization of gene transfer protocols--feasibility study in mice. Radiology. 2003 Sep;228(3):768-75.

[43] Satkauskas S, Bureau MF, Mahfoudi A, Mir LM. Slow accumulation of plasmid in muscle cells: supporting evidence for a mechanism of DNA uptake by receptor-mediated endocytosis. MolTher. 2001 Oct;4(4):317-23.

[44] Cappelletti M, Zampaglione I, Rizzuto G, Ciliberto G, La Monica N, Fattori E. Gene electro-transfer improves transduction by modifying the fate of intramuscular DNA. J Gene Med. 2003 Apr;5(4):324-32.

[45] Bureau MF, Naimi S, Torero Ibad R, Seguin J, Georger C, Arnould E, et al. Intramuscular plasmid DNA electrotransfer: biodistribution and degradation. BiochimBiophysActa. 2004 Jan 20;1676(2):138-48.

[46] Burgain A, Scherman D, Bigey P. Electrotransfert : concept et historique. L'Actualité-Chimique. 2009;327*328:68-74.

[47] Scheerlinck JP, Karlis J, Tjelle TE, Presidente PJ, Mathiesen I, Newton SE. In vivo electroporation improves immune responses to DNA vaccination in sheep. Vaccine. 2004 Apr 16;22(13-14):1820-5.

[48] Tollefsen S, Vordermeier M, Olsen I, Storset AK, Reitan LJ, Clifford D, et al. DNA injection in combination with electroporation: a novel method for vaccination of farmed ruminants. Scand J Immunol. 2003 Mar;57(3):229-38.

[49] Rambabu KM, Rao SH, Rao NM. Efficient expression of transgenes in adult zebrafish by electroporation. BMC Biotechnol. 2005;5:29.

[50] Miklavcic D, Semrov D, Mekid H, Mir LM. A validated model of in vivo electric field distribution in tissues for electrochemotherapy and for DNA electrotransfer for gene therapy. BiochimBiophysActa. 2000 Sep 1;1523(1):73-83.

[51] Bloquel C, Fabre E, Bureau MF, Scherman D. Plasmid DNA electrotransfer for intracellular and secreted proteins expression: new methodological developments and applications. J Gene Med. 2004 Feb;6Suppl 1:S11-23.

[52] Mathiesen I. Electropermeabilization of skeletal muscle enhances gene transfer in vivo. Gene Ther. 1999 Apr;6(4):508-14.

[53] Taylor J, Babbs CF, Alzghoul MB, Olsen A, Latour M, Pond AL, et al. Optimization of ectopic gene expression in skeletal muscle through DNA transfer by electroporation. BMC Biotechnol. 2004 May 18;4:11.

[54] Maccarrone M, Bladergroen MR, Rosato N, Finazzi Agro AF. Role of lipid peroxidation in electroporation-induced cell permeability. BiochemBiophys Res Commun. 1995 Apr 17;209(2):417-25.

[55] Hartikka J, Sukhu L, Buchner C, Hazard D, Bozoukova V, Margalith M, et al. Electroporation-facilitated delivery of plasmid DNA in skeletal muscle: plasmid dependence of muscle damage and effect of poloxamer 188. MolTher. 2001 Nov;4(5):407-15.

[56] Rubenstrunk A, Mahfoudi A, Scherman D. Delivery of electric pulses for DNA electrotransfer to mouse muscle does not induce the expression of stress related genes. Cell BiolToxicol. 2004 Feb;20(1):25-31.

[57] Trollet C, Scherman D, Bigey P. Delivery of DNA into muscle for treating systemic diseases: advantages and challenges. Methods Mol Biol. 2008;423:199-214.

[58] Schertzer JD, Lynch GS. Plasmid-based gene transfer in mouse skeletal muscle by electroporation. Methods Mol Biol. 2008;433:115-25.

[59]  Mennuni C, Calvaruso F, Zampaglione I, Rizzuto G, Rinaudo D, Dammassa E, et al. Hyaluronidase increases electrogene transfer efficiency in skeletal muscle. Hum Gene Ther. 2002 Feb 10;13(3):355-65.

[60]  Favre D, Cherel Y, Provost N, Blouin V, Ferry N, Moullier P, et al. Hyaluronidase enhances recombinant adeno-associated virus (rAAV)-mediated gene transfer in the rat skeletal muscle. Gene Ther. 2000 Aug;7(16):1417-20.

[61]  McMahon JM, Signori E, Wells KE, Fazio VM, Wells DJ. Optimisation of electrotransfer of plasmid into skeletal muscle by pretreatment with hyaluronidase -- increased expression with reduced muscle damage. Gene Ther. 2001 Aug;8(16):1264-70.

[62]  Davis HL, Whalen RG, Demeneix BA. Direct gene transfer into skeletal muscle in vivo: factors affecting efficiency of transfer and stability of expression. Hum Gene Ther. 1993 Apr;4(2):151-9.

[63]  Nicol F, Wong M, MacLaughlin FC, Perrard J, Wilson E, Nordstrom JL, et al. Poly-L-glutamate, an anionic polymer, enhances transgene expression for plasmids delivered by intramuscular injection with in vivo electroporation. Gene Ther. 2002 Oct; 9(20):1351-8.

[64]  Mir LM, Moller PH, Andre F, Gehl J. Electric pulse-mediated gene delivery to various animal tissues. Adv Genet. 2005;54:83-114.

[65]  Goldspink G. Skeletal muscle as an artificial endocrine tissue. Best Pract Res ClinEndocrinolMetab. 2003 Jun;17(2):211-22.

[66]  Escoffre JM, Debin A, Reynes JP, Drocourt D, Tiraby G, Hellaudais L, et al. Long-lasting in vivo gene silencing by electrotransfer of shRNA expressing plasmid. Technol Cancer Res Treat. 2008 Apr;7(2):109-16.

[67]  Kanitakis J. Anatomy, histology and immunohistochemistry of normal human skin. Eur J Dermatol. 2002 Jul-Aug;12(4):390-9; quiz 400-1.

[68]  Denet AR, Vanbever R, Preat V. Skin electroporation for transdermal and topical delivery. Adv Drug Deliv Rev. 2004 Mar 27;56(5):659-74.

[69]  Jadoul A, Bouwstra J, Preat VV. Effects of iontophoresis and electroporation on the stratum corneum. Review of the biophysical studies. Adv Drug Deliv Rev. 1999 Jan 4;35(1):89-105.

[70]  Pavselj N, Preat V. DNA electrotransfer into the skin using a combination of one high- and one low-voltage pulse. J Control Release. 2005 Sep 2;106(3):407-15.

[71]  Zhang L, Nolan E, Kreitschitz S, Rabussay DP. Enhanced delivery of naked DNA to the skin by non-invasive in vivo electroporation. BiochimBiophysActa. 2002 Aug 15;1572(1):1-9.

[72]  Dujardin N, Staes E, Kalia Y, Clarys P, Guy R, Preat V. In vivo assessment of skin electroporation using square wave pulses. J Control Release. 2002 Feb 19;79(1-3): 219-27.

[73] Cemazar M, Golzio M, Sersa G, Escoffre JM, Coer A, Vidic S, et al. Hyaluronidase and collagenase increase the transfection efficiency of gene electrotransfer in various murine tumors. Hum Gene Ther. 2012 Jan;23(1):128-37.

[74] Trollet C, Pereira Y, Burgain A, Litzler E, Mezrahi M, Seguin J, et al. Generation of high-titer neutralizing antibodies against botulinum toxins A, B, and E by DNA electrotransfer. Infect Immun. 2009 May;77(5):2221-9.

[75] Adachi O, Nakano A, Sato O, Kawamoto S, Tahara H, Toyoda N, et al. Gene transfer of Fc-fusion cytokine by in vivo electroporation: application to gene therapy for viral myocarditis. Gene Ther. 2002 May;9(9):577-83.

[76] Daud AI, DeConti RC, Andrews S, Urbas P, Riker AI, Sondak VK, et al. Phase I trial of interleukin-12 plasmid electroporation in patients with metastatic melanoma. J ClinOncol. 2008 Dec 20;26(36):5896-903.

[77] Heller LC, Heller R. Electroporation gene therapy preclinical and clinical trials for melanoma. Curr Gene Ther. 2010 Aug;10(4):312-7.

[78] Bettan M, Ivanov MA, Mir LM, Boissiere F, Delaere P, Scherman D. Efficient DNA electrotransfer into tumors. Bioelectrochemistry. 2000 Sep;52(1):83-90.

[79] Bloquel C, Bessis N, Boissier MC, Scherman D, Bigey P. Gene therapy of collagen-induced arthritis by electrotransfer of human tumor necrosis factor-alpha soluble receptor I variants. Hum Gene Ther. 2004 Feb;15(2):189-201.

[80] Gollins H, McMahon J, Wells KE, Wells DJ. High-efficiency plasmid gene transfer into dystrophic muscle. Gene Ther. 2003 Mar;10(6):504-12.

[81] Tanaka T, Ichimaru N, Takahara S, Yazawa K, Hatori M, Suzuki K, et al. In vivo gene transfer of hepatocyte growth factor to skeletal muscle prevents changes in rat kidneys after 5/6 nephrectomy. Am J Transplant. 2002 Oct;2(9):828-36.

[82] Bakker JM, Bleeker WK, Parren PW. Therapeutic antibody gene transfer: an active approach to passive immunity. MolTher. 2004 Sep;10(3):411-6.

[83] Perez N, Bigey P, Scherman D, Danos O, Piechaczyk M, Pelegrin M. Regulatable systemic production of monoclonal antibodies by in vivo muscle electroporation. Genet Vaccines Ther. 2004 Mar 23;2(1):2.

[84] Bernal SD, Ona ET, Riego-Javier A, R DEV, Cristal-Luna GR, Laguatan JB, et al. Anti-cancer immune reactivity and long-term survival after treatment of metastatic ovarian cancer with dendritic cells. OncolLett. Jan;3(1):66-74.

[85] Goto T, Nishi T, Kobayashi O, Tamura T, Dev SB, Takeshima H, et al. Combination electro-gene therapy using herpes virus thymidine kinase and interleukin-12 expression plasmids is highly efficient against murine carcinomas in vivo. MolTher. 2004 Nov;10(5):929-37.

[86] Shao D, Zeng Q, Fan Z, Li J, Zhang M, Zhang Y, et al. Monitoring HSV-TK/ganciclo-vir cancer suicide gene therapy using CdTe/CdS core/shell quantum dots. Biomateri-als. 2012 Jun;33(17):4336-44.

[87] Shibata MA, Morimoto J, Otsuki Y. Suppression of murine mammary carcinoma growth and metastasis by HSVtk/GCV gene therapy using in vivo electroporation. Cancer Gene Ther. 2002 Jan;9(1):16-27.

[88] Prabha S, Sharma B, Labhasetwar V. Inhibition of tumor angiogenesis and growth by nanoparticle-mediated p53 gene therapy in mice. Cancer Gene Ther. 2012 Aug;19(8): 530-7.

[89] Finetti F, Terzuoli E, Bocci E, Coletta I, Polenzani L, Mangano G, et al. Pharmacologi-cal inhibition of microsomal prostaglandin e synthase-1 suppresses epidermal growth factor receptor-mediated tumor growth and angiogenesis. PLoS One. 2012;7(7):e40576.

[90] Hanari N, Matsubara H, Hoshino I, Akutsu Y, Nishimori T, Murakami K, et al. Com-binatory gene therapy with electrotransfer of midkine promoter-HSV-TK and inter-leukin-21. Anticancer Res. 2007 Jul-Aug;27(4B):2305-10.

[91] Cemazar M, Jarm T, Sersa G. Cancer electrogene therapy with interleukin-12. Curr Gene Ther. 2010 Aug;10(4):300-11.

[92] Tamura T, Nishi T, Goto T, Takeshima H, Ushio Y, Sakata T. Combination of IL-12 and IL-18 of electro-gene therapy synergistically inhibits tumor growth. Anticancer Res. 2003 Mar-Apr;23(2B):1173-9.

[93] Craig R, Cutrera J, Zhu S, Xia X, Lee YH, Li S. Administering plasmid DNA encoding tumor vessel-anchored IFN-alpha for localizing gene product within or into tumors. MolTher. 2008 May;16(5):901-6.

[94] Zhang L, Zhao L, Zhao D, Lin G, Guo B, Li Y, et al. Inhibition of tumor growth and induction of apoptosis in prostate cancer cell lines by overexpression of tissue inhibi-tor of matrix metalloproteinase-3. Cancer Gene Ther. 2010 Mar;17(3):171-9.

[95] Zhu LP, Yin Y, Xing J, Li C, Kou L, Hu B, et al. Therapeutic efficacy of Bifidobacter-iumlongum-mediated human granulocyte colony-stimulating factor and/or endosta-tin combined with cyclophosphamide in mouse-transplanted tumors. Cancer Sci. 2009 Oct;100(10):1986-90.

[96] Chudley L, McCann K, Mander A, Tjelle T, Campos-Perez J, Godeseth R, et al. DNA fusion-gene vaccination in patients with prostate cancer induces high-frequency CD8(+) T-cell responses and increases PSA doubling time. Cancer ImmunolImmun-other. 2012 May 22;2012:22.

[97] Low L, Mander A, McCann K, Dearnaley D, Tjelle T, Mathiesen I, et al. DNA vacci-nation with electroporation induces increased antibody responses in patients with prostate cancer. Hum Gene Ther. 2009 Nov;20(11):1269-78.

[98]  Pichavant C, Chapdelaine P, Cerri DG, Bizario JC, Tremblay JP. Electrotransfer of the full-length dog dystrophin into mouse and dystrophic dog muscles. Hum Gene Ther. Nov;21(11):1591-601.

[99]  Kreiss P, Bettan M, Crouzet J, Scherman D. Erythropoietin secretion and physiological effect in mouse after intramuscular plasmid DNA electrotransfer. J Gene Med. 1999 Jul-Aug;1(4):245-50.

[100]  Rizzuto G, Cappelletti M, Maione D, Savino R, Lazzaro D, Costa P, et al. Efficient and regulated erythropoietin production by naked DNA injection and muscle electroporation. ProcNatlAcadSci U S A. 1999 May 25;96(11):6417-22.

[101]  Payen E, Bettan M, Henri A, Tomkiewitcz E, Houque A, Kuzniak I, et al. Oxygen tension and a pharmacological switch in the regulation of transgene expression for gene therapy. J Gene Med. 2001 Sep-Oct;3(5):498-504.

[102]  Payen E, Bettan M, Rouyer-Fessard P, Beuzard Y, Scherman D. Improvement of mouse beta-thalassemia by electrotransfer of erythropoietin cDNA. ExpHematol. 2001 Mar;29(3):295-300.

[103]  Dalle B, Henri A, Rouyer-Fessard P, Bettan M, Scherman D, Beuzard Y, et al. Dimeric erythropoietin fusion protein with enhanced erythropoietic activity in vitro and in vivo. Blood. 2001 Jun 15;97(12):3776-82.

[104]  Livnah O, Stura EA, Middleton SA, Johnson DL, Jolliffe LK, Wilson IA. Crystallographic evidence for preformed dimers of erythropoietin receptor before ligand activation. Science. 1999 Feb 12;283(5404):987-90.

[105]  Fabre EE, Bigey P, Beuzard Y, Scherman D, Payen E. Careful adjustment of Epo nonviral gene therapy for beta-thalassemicanaemia treatment. Genet Vaccines Ther. 2008;6:10.

[106]  Gothelf A, Hojman P, Gehl J. Therapeutic levels of erythropoietin (EPO) achieved after gene electrotransfer to skin in mice. Gene Ther. 2010 Sep;17(9):1077-84.

[107]  Marshall WG, Jr., Boone BA, Burgos JD, Gografe SI, Baldwin MK, Danielson ML, et al. Electroporation-mediated delivery of a naked DNA plasmid expressing VEGF to the porcine heart enhances protein expression. Gene Ther. 2010 Mar;17(3):419-23.

[108]  Ayuni EL, Gazdhar A, Giraud MN, Kadner A, Gugger M, Cecchini M, et al. In vivo electroporation mediated gene delivery to the beating heart. PLoS One. 2010;5(12):e14467.

[109]  Dean D. DNA electrotransfer to the skin: a highly translatable approach to treat peripheral artery disease. Gene Ther. 2010 Jun;17(6):691.

[110]  Bloquel C, Bejjani R, Bigey P, Bedioui F, Doat M, BenEzra D, et al. Plasmid electrotransfer of eye ciliary muscle: principles and therapeutic efficacy using hTNF-alpha soluble receptor in uveitis. Faseb J. 2006 Feb;20(2):389-91.

[111] Touchard E, Bloquel C, Bigey P, Kowalczuk L, Jonet L, Thillaye-Goldenberg B, et al. Effects of ciliary muscle plasmid electrotransfer of TNF-alpha soluble receptor variants in experimental uveitis. Gene Ther. 2009 Jul;16(7):862-73.

[112] Touchard E, Berdugo M, Bigey P, El Sanharawi M, Savoldelli M, Naud MC, et al. SuprachoroidalElectrotransfer: A Nonviral Gene Delivery Method to Transfect the Choroid and the Retina Without Detaching the Retina. MolTher. 2012 Jan 17.

[113] Hojman P, Brolin C, Gissel H, Brandt C, Zerahn B, Pedersen BK, et al. Erythropoietin over-expression protects against diet-induced obesity in mice through increased fat oxidation in muscles. PLoS One. 2009;4(6):e5894.

[114] Bruce CR, Hoy AJ, Turner N, Watt MJ, Allen TL, Carpenter K, et al. Overexpression of carnitine palmitoyltransferase-1 in skeletal muscle is sufficient to enhance fatty acid oxidation and improve high-fat diet-induced insulin resistance. Diabetes. 2009 Mar;58(3):550-8.

[115] Kanzleiter T, Preston E, Wilks D, Ho B, Benrick A, Reznick J, et al. Overexpression of the orphan receptor Nur77 alters glucose metabolism in rat muscle cells and rat muscle in vivo. Diabetologia. 2010 Jun;53(6):1174-83.

[116] Quinn A, Jiang W, Velaz-Faircloth M, Cobb AJ, Henry SC, Frothingham R. In vivo protein expression and immune responses generated by DNA vaccines expressing mycobacterial antigens fused with a reporter protein. Vaccine. 2002 Aug 19;20(25-26): 3187-92.

[117] Kirman JR, Seder RA. DNA vaccination: the answer to stable, protective T-cell memory? CurrOpinImmunol. 2003 Aug;15(4):471-6.

[118] Widera G, Austin M, Rabussay D, Goldbeck C, Barnett SW, Chen M, et al. Increased DNA vaccine delivery and immunogenicity by electroporation in vivo. J Immunol. 2000 May 1;164(9):4635-40.

[119] Zucchelli S, Capone S, Fattori E, Folgori A, Di Marco A, Casimiro D, et al. Enhancing B- and T-cell immune response to a hepatitis C virus E2 DNA vaccine by intramuscular electrical gene transfer. J Virol. 2000 Dec;74(24):11598-607.

[120] Tollefsen S, Tjelle T, Schneider J, Harboe M, Wiker H, Hewinson G, et al. Improved cellular and humoral immune responses against Mycobacterium tuberculosis antigens after intramuscular DNA immunisation combined with muscle electroporation. Vaccine. 2002 Sep 10;20(27-28):3370-8.

[121] Bachy M, Boudet F, Bureau M, Girerd-Chambaz Y, Wils P, Scherman D, et al. Electric pulses increase the immunogenicity of an influenza DNA vaccine injected intramuscularly in the mouse. Vaccine. 2001 Feb 8;19(13-14):1688-93.

[122] Tjelle TE, Corthay A, Lunde E, Sandlie I, Michaelsen TE, Mathiesen I, et al. Monoclonal antibodies produced by muscle after plasmid injection and electroporation. MolTher. 2004 Mar;9(3):328-36.

# siRNA and Gene Formulation for Efficient Gene Therapy

Ian S. Blagbrough and Abdelkader A. Metwally

Additional information is available at the end of the chapter

## 1. Introduction

Whilst small interfering RNA (siRNA, also known as short interfering RNA) has a somewhat chequered history with regard to its discovery and initial usage, the "mammalian" research community singularly neither reading nor citing the output from the "plant" research community, it is now recognised in terms of $bn being invested and spent that RNA interference (RNAi), sequence specific post-transcriptional gene silencing (PTGS) by siRNA, has many potential therapeutic applications [1] as well as being an important tool in the study of functional genomics. The site and mechanism of action of siRNA requires that these short double-stranded nucleic acids are delivered to the cytosol of target cells. Therefore, formulation is required in a strategy similar to that for gene therapy, although not requiring access to the nucleus. Efficient medicines design should come with an understanding of the problem at the molecular level. Our contributions are aimed at the use of non-viral gene therapy and this Chapter therefore has such a focus.

## 2. RNA interference

### 2.1. History and mechanism of RNA interference

siRNA is a double-stranded RNA (dsRNA) typically of 21-25 nucleotides per strand. siRNA operates as a part of the cellular mechanism called RNAi, which was first noticed in petunia flowers (*Petunia hybrida*) which showed reduced pigmentation on the introduction of exogenous genes that were meant to increase pigmentation [2, 3]. These experiments aimed at increasing the pigmentation of the petunia flowers by means of introducing additional gene constructs expressing either chalcone synthase [2, 3] or dihydroflavonol-4-reductase [2]. However, the resultant plants produced completely white flowers and/or flowers with white or pale sectors on a pigmented background. The exact mechanism was not identified at the time and was simply termed co-suppression. The transcription level of the suppressed chalcone synthase genes in petunia flowers was found to be similar to that of the non-suppressed genes, and thus the co-suppression must have been at the post-transcriptional level [4]. Later in 1997, the suppression of chalcone synthase endogene in petunia flowers was suggested to be related to formation of RNA duplexes by intermolecular pairing of complementary sequences between the coding sequence and the 3'-UTR sequence of the transgene mRNA [5]. Indeed, the seminal contributions the plant RNAi community have made to this RNAi field are also reflected in the research of Hamilton and Sir David C. Baulcombe in the Sainsbury Laboratory, Norwich, UK, on PTGS as a nucleotide sequence-specific defence mechanism that can target both cellular and viral mRNAs with RNA molecules of a uniform length, ~25 nucleotides [6]. That RNA silencing involves the processing of dsRNA into 21-26 long siRNA to mediate gene suppression (correspondingly complementary to the dsRNA) was demonstrated in Arabidopsis, "RNA silencing pathways in plants that may also apply in animals" [7]. That Arabidopsis ARGONAUTE1 RNA-binding protein is an RNA slicer that selectively recruits microRNAs and siRNAs was shown to be by a key mechanism similar to but different from that found in animals [8]. In 1998, Fire, Mello and co-workers reported the reduction or inhibition (hence genetic "interference") of the expression of the *unc-22* gene *in Caenorhabditis elegans* by means of dsRNA that is homologous to 742 nucleotides in the targeted gene [9], a discovery that was awarded the Nobel Prize in medicine or physiology in 2006. The target gene expresses an abundant although nonessential myofilament protein. Decreasing *unc-22* activity resulted in an increasingly severe twitching phenotype, while complete inhibition resulted in impaired motility and muscle structural defects. The target gene inhibition was best achieved with dsRNA, while using the individual sense or anti-sense RNA strands resulted only in modest silencing. The authors also noticed that only few copies of the dsRNA are required per cell to initiate a potent and specific response, rejecting the hypothesis that the mechanism of interaction with target gene mRNA is stoichiometric in nature, and thus the role of the dsRNA in the interference machinery must be catalytic or amplifying.

Elbashir et al. reported in 2001 that sequence-specific gene silencing of endogenous and heterologous genes with 21 nucleotide siRNA occurs in mammalian cell cultures [10]. The reporter genes coding for sea pansy (*Renilla reniformis*) and firefly (*Photinus pyralis*) luciferases were silenced successfully in different cell lines including human embryonic kidney cells (293) and the cervix cancer cells (HeLa cell line, the first human cell line grown in vitro with success [11]), as well as the endogenous gene coding for the nuclear envelope proteins lamin A and lamin C in HeLa cells. The authors used dsRNA of length 21 or 22 nucleotides with 3'-symmetrical 2-nucleotide overhangs on each strand, as dsRNA with length >30 nucleotides initiates an immune response e.g. inducing interferon synthesis) that leads to non-specific mRNA degradation, which was evident from non-specific silencing of luciferase with 50 and 500 nucleotides dsRNA in HeLa S3 cells, COS-7 cells (kidney cells of the African green monkey), and NIH/3T3 cells (mouse fibroblasts) [10]. The RNAi mechanism of action continues to be investigated in detail and reviewed thoroughly [12-17]. The RNAi mechanism involves the incorporation of dsRNA segments (e.g. siRNA) that have a sequence complementary to the targeted mRNA in a protein complex. This core complex which carries-out mRNA degradation is the RNA induced silencing complex (RISC) [18-20]. The degradation process requires the key argonaute family of proteins, which contain a domain with RNase H (endonuclease) type of activity that catalyse cleavage of the phosphodiester bonds of the targeted mRNA. RISC assembly and subsequently its function to mediate sequence specific mRNA degradation occur in the cytoplasm of the cell [16]. The source of the dsRNA segments incorporated in RISC can be endogenously processed microRNA (miRNA), short hairpin RNA (shRNA), or synthetic siRNA. miRNA is produced from endogenous DNA through the action of RNA polymerase II resulting in the formation of non-coding RNA called primary miRNA (pri-miRNA), which is processed in the nucleus by a protein complex containing an enzyme known as Drosha and a dsRNA binding protein cofactor called Pasha (DGCR8). Drosha cleaves pri-miRNA to produce (pre-miRNA), a dsRNA of 70-90 nucleotides and having a hairpin loop, which binds to Exportin 5 protein and is transferred from the nucleus into the cytoplasm. Pre-miRNA is processed by Dicer (RNase III enzyme) in the cytoplasm to give miRNA, typically of 22 nucleotides in length and having two nucleotide overhangs at the 3'-position [16, 21], shRNA is produced by transcription from an exogenous DNA that is delivered to the nucleus, and codes for a hairpin shaped RNA with segments of length 19-29 nucleotides and loop of 9 nucleotides [22, 23] which can then be processed by Dicer and incorporated in the RNAi machinery.

Once in the cytoplasm, the processed dsRNA (miRNA, processed shRNA, or siRNA) is then incorporated into a protein complex (RISC-loading complex, RLC). In *Drosophila* the RLC is composed of the dsRNA, heterodimer protein DCR2 (Dicer variant)/R2D2, possibly including the catalytic argonaute proteins as well in this complex. The active RISC is formed when one of the RNA strands in the complex is cleaved (the passenger strand) and the strand with the less thermodynamic stable 5'-end (guide/anti-sense strand) remains in the complex. The mRNA with complementary sequence to the guide strand binds to the active RISC and is cleaved by the endoribonuclease activity of the argonaute component of the complex (Figure 1).

## 2.2. RNA duplex structure

RNA is a polymer of ribonucleotides. Each RNA nucleotide is composed of one nucleobase, the monosaccharide pentose ribose, and one phosphate group. The nucleobases in RNA are adenine (purine base), guanine (purine base), uracil (pyrimidine base), and cytosine (pyrimidine base) (Figure 2). A nucleoside is formed when each base is connected via a glycosidic bond to the anomeric carbon 1' of ribose, thus when glycosylated, adenine, guanine, uracil, and cytosine nucleobases give adenosine, guanosine, uridine, and cytidine nucleosides. Each two nucleosides are connected via a phosphate diester bond between the 3' of one nucleoside and 5' of the next nucleoside to form the RNA polynucleotide strand. The main differences in the primary structure of RNA and DNA are that RNA pentose is ribose while DNA pentose is 2'-deoxyribose, and the RNA incorporates the nucleobase uracil instead of thymine.

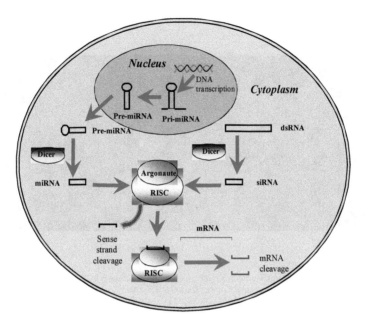

**Figure 1.** RNAi mechanism in a eukaryotic cell. The source of the antisense strand incorporated in RISC can be miRNA, processed exogenous long dsRNA, or synthetic siRNA delivered to the cell.

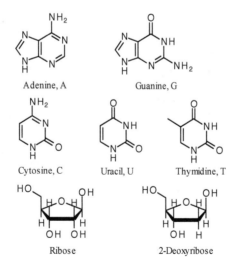

**Figure 2.** Nucleobases and pentoses of RNA and DNA.

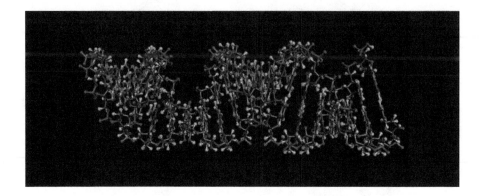

**Figure 3.** siRNA duplex 22-mer targeting the enhanced green fluorescent protein (EGFP) mRNA. The two deoxythymi-dine residues at the 3'-end of the sense strand are not shown. Sense strand: 5'-GCAAGCUGACCCUGAAGUUCAUTT-3' Anti-sense strand: 5'-AUGAACUUCAGGGUCAGCUUGCCG-3' Target DNA sequence: 5'-CGGCAAGCTGACCCTGAAGTT-CAT-3'

In order to form an RNA duplex (Figure 3), the strands with complementary nucleotide sequence bind together by hydrogen bonds. Adenine is bound to uracil with two hydrogen bonds while guanine is bound to cytosine with three hydrogen bonds, thus forming what is known as Watson-Crick base pairs. RNA duplexes under normal physiological conditions are in the form of A-helix. This type of duplex is a right-handed helix [24-26].

The presence of the 2'-hydroxyl group of the ribose and the lack of the methyl group on the nucleotide uridine (in contrast to the methylated thymidine) results in structural differences between RNA and DNA, with the 2'-hydroxyl group of RNA being the major cause of the differences. The sugar phosphate backbone of RNA duplexes is stabilized by the 2'-hydroxyl in the C3'-endo position, while DNA adopts the C2'-endo position (Figure 4). Thus, the RNA duplex takes the A-helix form while the DNA helix takes the B-form. The A-helix form is suggested to have a greater hydration shell, giving RNA duplexes more thermodynamic stability and more rigidity compared to DNA duplexes [24-26]. RNA A-helix completes one complete rotation in 11-12 base pair (bp) compared to 10 bp for DNA, with a rise of 2.7 Å per bp of RNA [27]. The A-helix geometry has been suggested to be the major factor explaining why dsRNA and not dsDNA is involved in the RNAi machinery [28], where the A-helix geometry between the guide strand and the complementary target mRNA is essential for the catalytic activity of the argonaute 2 protein in the RISC.

As a result of the presence of a hydroxyl group in the 2'-position of the ribose in the RNA backbone, the RNA phosphodiester backbone is more susceptible to hydrolysis by nucleases compared to the DNA which lacks the 2'-hydroxyl in its 2'-deoxyribose [29]. Incubation of

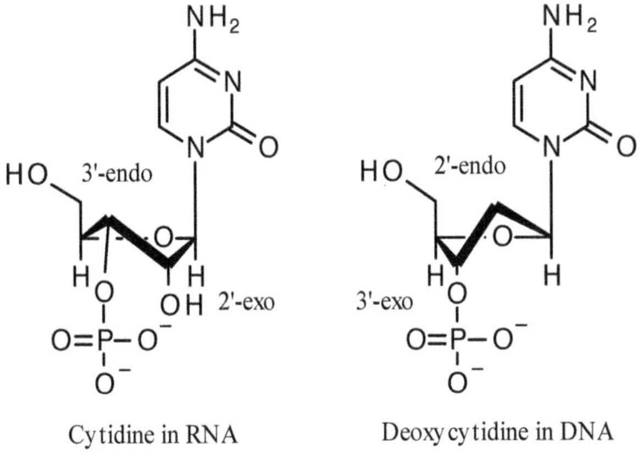

**Figure 4.** 3'-endo ribose configuration of RNA (left) vs 2'-endo (right) of 2'-deoxyribose in DNA. Shown is cytidine (RNA) and deoxycytidine (DNA) with the 3'-hydroxyl phosphorylated. The hydrogen atoms at C2' and C3' are not displayed for clarity.

siRNA in fetal bovine or human serum at 37 °C resulted in the degradation and partial or complete loss of activity [30]. When incubated in human plasma at 37 °C, more than 50% of the unmodified siRNA was degraded within one minute, and practically all siRNA was completely degraded within 4 hours [31]. Although Ribonuclease A (RNase A, an endoribonuclease) cleaves single stranded RNA, siRNA degradation in serum was reported to be mainly due to RNase-like activity[32], which is suggested to occur during transient breaking of the hydrogen bonds joining the two siRNA strands. In addition to the RNase A family of enzymes, blood serum contains phosphatases and exoribonucleases which can also affect degradation of siRNA at nuclease-sensitive sites on both strands [33].

## 2.3. Therapeutic potential of RNAi based therapies

RNAi based therapies emerged in the period following its discovery in 1998 in plants, and are promising therapeutic candidates to treat various types of diseases, ranging from age related macular oedema to respiratory tract infections to various types of cancer [34-36]. In addition to siRNA based therapies, shRNA [37, 38] and miRNA [39] are potential therapeutic tools. siRNA based therapeutics are already in phase I and phase II clinical trials; representative examples of clinical trials involving siRNA are shown in Table 1. The basic concept is the reduction or inhibition of the expression of a protein that is involved in the pathophysiological pathway of the target disease (silencing/knocking-down the target gene). This concept is evident from using Cand5 siRNA targeting the mRNA translating the vascular endothelial growth factor (VEGF), thus reducing/inhibiting angiogenesis and preventing progression of wet age related macular oedema (Table 1) [40]. Atu027 siRNA targets the biosynthesis of protein kinase N3 which plays a role in cancer metastasis [41].

| siRNA | Disease | Vector/ Route | Phase | Sponsor |
|---|---|---|---|---|
| Cand5/ Bevasiranib | Diabetic macular oedema | None/ Intravitreal | Phase II | Opko Health (Miami, USA) |
| Cand5/ Bevasiranib | Age-related macular degeneration | None/ Intravitreal | Phase II (Phase III halted) | Opko Health (Miami, USA) |
| ALN-RSV01 | Respiratory syncytial virus infection | None/ Intranasal | Phase II | Alnylam Pharmaceuticals (Cambridge, USA) |
| CALAA-01 | Solid tumour/melanoma | Cyclodextrin nanoparticles/ Intravenous | Phase I | Calando (Pasadena, CA, USA) |
| Atu027 | Colorectal cancer metastasizing to the liver | AtuPlex-Liposome/ Intravenous | Phase I | Silence Therapeutics (London, UK) |
| Two siRNA against TGFBI and COX-2 STP705 | Wound healing | Nanoparticles/ Intravenous | Phase I | Sirnaomics (Gaithersburg, MD, USA) |
| I5NP | Protection from acute kidney injury after cardiac bypass surgery | None/ Intravenous | Phase I | Quark Pharmaceuticals (Fremont, USA) |
| TKM-080301 | Against PLK1 gene product in patients with hepatic cancer | Lipid nanoparticles/ Hepatic intra-arterial administration | Phase I | NCI (Maryland, USA) |

**Table 1.** Representative clinical trials using siRNA (http://clinicaltrials.gov/ct2/home, accessed on 5/8/2012).

The therapeutic application of siRNA requires overcoming several barriers (Figure 5) for its intracellular delivery and the subsequent functional gene silencing activity [42-44]. Those barriers are mainly due to siRNA specific characteristics, most important are having a highly negative charge due to their phosphate backbone (on average 40-50 negative charges per siRNA), being susceptible to degradation by nucleases, and having relatively large molecular weight (13-15 kDa) compared to conventional small drug molecules. First, local delivery (such as intravitreal) is different from intravenous delivery, where the latter will subject the siRNA to the serum ribonucleases, which results in degrading non-modified siRNA within time periods that vary from minutes to hours [31]. siRNA injected intravenously in rats was reported to be cleared rapidly from circulation and accumulates in kidneys within minutes of injection [45], making it useful only if the target organ is the kidney.

In order to gain access into the cytoplasm where siRNA can exert its biological activity, the polyribonucleotide must pass first through the interstitial space then through the target cell membrane. This will be a difficult task, since both the extracellular matrix in many tissue types and the cell membrane incorporate negatively charged glycosaminoglycans (e.g. heparan sulfate) [46]. In addition, cell membranes contain negatively charged phospholipids (e.g. phosphatidyl serine) therefore the membrane is negatively charged [46, 47]. The net result is an unfavourable repulsive interaction with naked siRNA. As a result, different strategies are being developed to overcome the barriers to reproducible and functional siRNA delivery, and these approaches fall into two general categories. One category is modifying the siRNA, the other is deploying a vector to protect the siRNA and increase its efficiency of delivery.

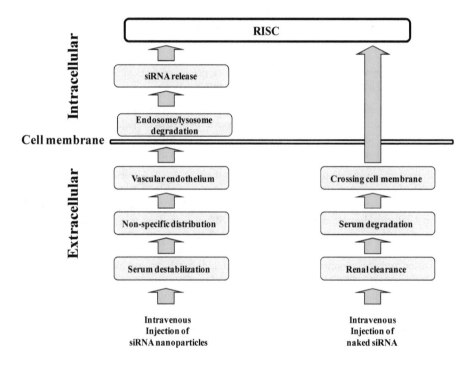

**Figure 5.** Summary of barriers to successful gene-silencing mediated by siRNA after intravenous injection, whether delivered naked or incorporated in nanoparticles.

## 3. Strategies to achieve efficient siRNA delivery and gene silencing

### 3.1. siRNA modifications

siRNA modifications include those carried out at the ribose residue, at the phosphate back-bone, at the RNA nucleotides, the siRNA termini, and/or by conjugation of other molecules to the siRNA molecule. Modifications to the ribose at the 2'-position are common [48], and include 2'-O-alkylation (e.g. 2'-O-methyl and 2'-O-methylethoxy) modifications. 2'-Fluoro RNA is another common modification. Locked nucleic acids (LNAs) have a methylene bridge connecting the 2'-$O$ to the 4'-C of the ribose unit, locking the sugar in the 3'-endo conformation. These modifications led to increased ribonuclease resistance [48, 49]. Modifications at the phosphate backbone include phosphorthioate, boranophosphate, and methylphosphonate linkages [48, 49] and is reported to increase siRNA stability against various ribonucleases and phophodiesterases [50]. siRNA nucleotides can be substituted with DNA nucleotides to increase stability and/or decrease unwanted siRNA off-target effects [51]. Modifications of the 3'-overhangs (usually two nucleotides in length) include incorporating deoxyribonucleotides to reduce costs and increase stability towards 3-exoribonucleases. The 5'-terminus chemical phosphorylation of the antisense strand results in higher gene silencing efficiency, while blunt ended duplexes were reported to be more resistant to exonucleases. The advantages of each of the aforementioned techniques, other modification strategies, as well as the considerations related to the degree of modification and its effect on gene silencing efficiency and associated cytotoxic effects have been reviewed thoroughly [48, 52-54].

The conjugation of drug molecules, aptamers, lipids, polymers, and peptides/proteins to siRNA could enhance in vivo delivery [55]. The main aims of such conjugations are: to enhance siRNA stability, increase in vivo half-life, control biodistribution, increase efficiency of intracellular delivery, while maintaining the gene silencing activity.

One strategy is to increase the hydrophobicity of the siRNA. Cholesterol was conjugated to the 5'-terminus of siRNA, the cholesterol-siRNA conjugate (chol-siRNA) resulted in better intracellular delivery compared to unmodified siRNA and retained gene silencing activity in vitro in $\beta$-galactosidase expressing liver cells [56]. When cholesterol was conjugated to the 3'-terminus of the sense (passenger) strand of siRNA, the conjugate had improved in vivo pharmacokinetics as the intravenous administration of chol-siRNA in mice resulted in its distribution and detection in the fat tissues, heart, kidneys, liver, and lungs, even 24 h after intravenous injection [57]. No significant amounts of unmodified siRNA were detected in the tissues 24 h after the intravenous injection. Conjugation of siRNA to bile acids and long-chain fatty acids, in addition to cholesterol, mediates siRNA uptake into cells and gene silencing in vivo [58]. The medium chain fatty-acid conjugates, namely lauroyl (C12), myristoyl (C14) and palmitoyl (C16), did not silence the target apolipoprotein B mRNA levels in mouse livers after intravenous injection. However, siRNA fatty-acid conjugates having long saturated chains, stearoyl (C18) and docosanoyl (C22), significantly reduced apolipoprotein B mRNA levels.

Cell penetrating peptides (CPPs) are used to facilitate cellular membrane crossing of many molecules displaying various properties such as antisense oligonucleotides, peptides, and proteins and are already being tested in vivo [59]. siRNA was conjugated to penetratin and transportin, to silence luciferase and green fluorescent protein (GFP) in different types of mammalian cells [60]. However, in vivo lung delivery in mouse of siRNA conjugated to penetratin and TAT(48-60), targeting p38 MAP kinase mRNA showed that the reduction in gene expression was peptide induced and the penetratin conjugated siRNA resulted in innate immunity response [61].

siRNA functioning against the VEGF mRNA was conjugated to poly(ethylene glycol) (PEG, 25 kDa) via a disulfide bond at the 3'-terminus of the sense strand [62]. The siRNA-PEG conjugate formed polyelectrolyte complex (PEC) micelles by electrostatic interaction with the cationic polymer polyethylenimine (PEI). The formed VEGF siRNA-PEG/PEI PEC micelles showed enhanced stability against nuclease degradation compared to the unmodified siRNA. These micelles efficiently silenced VEGF gene expression in prostate carcinoma cells (PC-3) and showed superior VEGF gene silencing compared to VEGF siRNA/PEI complexes in the presence of serum. PEG conjugation on its own enhanced the stability of the siRNA in serum containing medium. The prolonged stability of the PEC micelles was suggested to be due to the presence of PEG chains in the outer micellar shell layer, thus sterically hindering nuclease access into the siRNA in the micelle core [62]. Targeting molecules such as antibodies [63] and aptamers (peptides or single stranded DNA or RNA that have selective affinities toward target proteins) [64] have also been conjugated to siRNA, with the aim of increasing the efficiency of siRNA delivery to the target tissues.

Conjugating molecules to siRNA requires specific considerations. First, the site of conjugation (3'- and/or 5'-terminus, on sense and/or antisense strand) should be chosen such that it does not affect the activity of the siRNA and its ability to be incorporated in the RISC, or its ability to bind the target mRNA in the correct helix conformation. Second, the conjugated siRNA might have new properties that were not present in the unmodified parent siRNA. An example is the in vivo immune response resulting from the penetratin-siRNA conjugate [61]. Third, the conjugation process is multi-step, and the chemical reaction intermediates and products require efficient purification in order to meet the specifications of in vivo applications. These steps need to be repeated for each siRNA under investigation, which can be costly and time consuming. Thus, although there are clear advantages to synthesize siRNA conjugates, there are also disadvantages, and conjugation is therefore only one of two valuable approaches in the toolbox for preparing siRNA based therapies. The other valuable tool is complexation or incorporating the siRNA in a vector.

### 3.2. Viral vectors for shRNA delivery

Vectors for RNAi based therapies are either viral or non-viral vectors. Viral vectors (Table 2) are used to deliver genes encoding hairpin RNA structures such as shRNA and miRNA, which are then processed by the cellular RNAi machinery to the functional silencing dsRNA [65, 66].

Viral vectors offer two main advantages, the first is the very high efficiency compared to non-viral vectors [68], which can reach few orders of magnitude more than that achieved with non-viral vectors, and the second is the potential of long term expression of the delivered RNAi therapeutic, which is very useful in the treatment of chronic diseases such as HIV infection and viral hepatitis [69, 70]. Retroviruses are enveloped, single stranded RNA viruses and have a genome capacity of 7-10 kilobases (kb). They preferentially target dividing cells which limits their use to mitotic tissues (thus for example excluding brain and neurons). Retroviruses integrate their DNA in the host genome using an integrase enzyme, which provides the advantage of stable long term expression of the delivered transgene in the host cell and its descendants. However, integrating new DNA sequences into host genome carries the risk of

| | | Retrovirus/ Lentivirus | Adenovirus | Adeno-associated virus | Herpes virus |
|---|---|---|---|---|---|
| **Viral vector properties** | **Genome** | ssRNA | dsDNA | ssDNA | dsDNA |
| | **Capsid** | Icosahedral | Icosahedral | Icosahedral | Icosahedral |
| | **Envelope** | Enveloped | None | None | Enveloped |
| | **Viral Polymerase** | Positive | Negative | Negative | Negative |
| | **Diameter (nm)** | 80-130 | 70-90 | 18-26 | 150-200 |
| | **Genome size (kb)** | 7-10 | 38 | 5 | 120-200 |
| **Gene therapy related** | **Infection tropism** | Dividing* | Dividing/ Non-dividing | Dividing/ Non-dividing | Dividing/ Non-dividing |
| | **Virus genome integration** | Integrating | Non-integrating | Integrating | Non-integrating |
| | **Transgene expression** | Lasting | Transient | Lasting | Transient |
| | **Packaging capacity (kb)** | 7-8 | 8 | 4.5 | >30 |

* Lentiviral vectors can infect non-dividing cells as their pre-integration complex can traverse the nuclear membrane pores (NMP), in contrast to retrovirus pre-integration complex which does not traverse NMP, requiring the host-cell division to integrate the retroviral genome [67].

**Table 2.** Summary of properties of viral vectors that are commonly used in gene therapy (adapted from http:// www.genetherapynet.com/viral-vectors.html, accessed on 5/8/2012).

insertional mutagenesis [68, 71]. shRNA expression cassette delivered by a retroviral vector was used in rats to silence a RAS oncogene in order to suppress tumour growth [72]. Herpes virus was used successfully to deliver shRNA targeting exogenous $\beta$-galactosidase or endogenous trpv1 gene mRNA in the peripheral neurons in mice by injecting once directly into the sciatic nerve of the animals [73].

Unlike other retroviruses, lentiviruses can infect dividing as well as differentiated and non-dividing cells. The lentiviral genome can accommodate 7.5 kb [66], and their genome is integrated in the host cell genome, lentiviral vectors are generally preferred for long-term expression of transgenes, and efficient delivery in vivo to the brain, eye, and liver to induce long-term transgene expression as reported [74]. A lentiviral vector was used to deliver shRNA targeting Smad3 gene mRNA, and enhanced myogenesis of old and injured muscles [75].

Adenoviruses are non-enveloped viruses, with linear double stranded DNA. They preferably infect the upper respiratory tract and the ocular tissue. Their genome can accommodate up to 8 kb which can be extended to ≥25 kb in modified viruses that have their viral genes deleted [68]. These viruses can infect post mitotic cells and thus are good candidates for neurological diseases. Unless delivering genes that can exist as episomes in host cells, adenoviruses result only in transient expression of their cargo. However, although the host cells with the episome can express the delivered genes for the cell life time, these cells will eventually be removed by the host immune system [68]. shRNA targeting VEGF that was delivered by an adenoviral vector resulted in potent inhibition of angiogenesis and tumour growth in mice [76].

Adeno-associated virus (AAV) is a single stranded DNA non-pathogenic virus that can accommodate a 4.7 kb genome. They can infect dividing or non-dividing cells. The replication of AAV requires co-infection with adenovirus. The viral genome integrates into the host cell genome at a specific location on chromosome 19 [68]. Direct intracerebellar injection in a mouse model of spinocerebellar ataxia of an AAV vector delivering a cargo expressing shRNA targeting polyglutamine induced neurodegeneration significantly restored cerebellar morphology and improved motor coordination in mice [77].

Although highly efficient in delivering their cargo, viral vectors have their disadvantages. Adenoviral vectors have the disadvantage of triggering a strong immune (adaptive and innate) response by repeated administration, in addition to target organ immunotoxicity, specially hepatotoxicity [78-80], which resulted in 1999 in the death of one 18-year-old male who received high dose of adenovirus that was delivered directly in the hepatic artery in a clinical gene therapy safety study [81]. Clonal T-cell acute lymphoblastic leukemia caused by insertional mutagenesis in a gene therapy completed clinical trial involving patients suffering X-linked severe combined immunodeficiency (SCID-X1) was reported in one out of the 10 patients using a retroviral vector [82]. Integration of the vector genome material in the antisense orientation 35 kb upstream of the protooncogene (LMO2) caused over expression of the gene in the leukemic cells. In a similar study, 4 out of 9 patients developed leukemia within 3-6 years post-treatment mainly due to vector-mediated upregulation of host cellular oncogenes [83, 84]. In addition, immune responses (whether adaptive or innate) of varying degrees depending on the type of vector, dose, and target organs were reported for lentiviral, adenoviral, adeno-associated viral vectors [80].

Current research on viral vectors for gene therapy is focussed on approaches such as vector engineering e.g. modifying the viral capsid or pseuodotyping the envelope, different delivery strategies, and administration to immune-privileged sites that can tolerate the delivered viral vectors without responding with an inflammatory response [80, 85]. Other research focusses on the essential scaling-up process of vector production and increasing the packaging efficiency of the vectors [85], the processes without which, the wide spread and successful therapeutic use of the viral vectors will be very difficult to achieve.

### 3.3. Non-viral vectors

Non-viral vectors for gene and siRNA delivery are an alternative to viral vectors, as they do not suffer many of the disadvantages of the viral vectors, especially immunogenicity and tumourigenicity. The non-viral vectors can be classified generally as peptides, polymeric based vectors, carbohydrate based, and lipid based [86]. CPPs, also known as peptide transduction domains (PTDs), have shown the ability to cross the cellular membrane despite their relatively high molecular weight and size (Table 3).

PTDs generally are short amphipathic and/or cationic peptides that can transport many hydrophilic molecules across the cell membrane. A wide range of molecules including liposomes [87, 88], peptides, proteins [89], peptide nucleic acids [90] and polynucleotides [91] are delivered intracellularly using PTDs and they have also been applied in vivo [59, 92, 93].

| CPP | Sequence of CPP | Type of association with siRNA | Target mRNA |
|---|---|---|---|
| CADY | GLWRALWRLLRSLWRLLWRA | Non-covalent | GAPDH, p53 [94] |
| EB1 | LIRLWSHLIHIWFQNRRLKWKKK | Non-covalent | Luc [95] |
| MPG | GALFLGFLGAAGSTMGAWSQPKKKRKV | Non-covalent | Luc, GAPDH [96] Oct-3/4 [97] |
| Poly-arginine | RRRRRRRRR | Non-covalent | VEGF [98] |
| Penetratin | RQIKIWFQNRRMKWKK | Covalent | Luciferase (Luc), EGFP [60] |
| | | Covalent | SOD1, caspase-3 [99] |
| | | Covalent | Luc, p38 MAP kinase [61, 100] |
| Transportan | LIKKALAALAKLNIKLLYGASNLTWG | Covalent | Luc, EGFP [100] |
| TAT | GRKKRRQRRRPPQ | Covalent | EGFP, CDK9 [101] |

**Table 3.** Selected CPPs used for siRNA delivery [59].

It was reported by Frankel and Pabo in 1988 that the HIV-1 derived TAT protein could be taken up by cells growing in tissue culture [102], and that a small basic region of TAT (48-60) was essential for uptake by the cells [103]. PTDs include antennapedia homeodomain protein (Antp, penetratin), mitogen-activated protein (MAP), poly-arginine, transportan, VP22 [59, 92]. Two major pathways are involved in the uptake of PTDs and PTD-cargos: direct translocation at 4 °C and 37 °C and endocytosis-translocation at 37 °C. These mechanisms depend on many factors: cargo size, cell line, PTD concentration, and the type of PTD [59, 104, 105]. siRNA can be conjugated covalently to the CPP or can be complexed with the cationic groups of basic amino acids that are present in the backbone of the CPP. As a representative example of non-covalent complexation, CADY [94], which is basic due to its five arginine residues can complex with the negatively charged siRNA. Another example of non-covalent complexation is the poly-arginine CPP [98].

PEI (Figure 6) is an efficient, but toxic, plasmid DNA delivery vector. However, as a siRNA delivery vector PEI is reported to be much less efficient [106, 107]. This decreased efficiency is due to the dissociation of the siRNA/PEI complex upon interaction with the negatively charged cell membrane, which is suggested to be because of the short length of siRNA and the associated weak electrostatic interaction with PEI [108, 109]. Another drawback of PEI is its relatively high toxicity [110]. Thus, in addition to linear PEI, PEI polymers with a wide range of molecular weights were developed to increase PEI efficiency and/or decrease toxicity, although not all PEI are suitable for siRNA delivery [111]. The main advantage of PEI is the ability of its variety of amino groups to be protonated at lower pH (inside endosomes) leading to what is known as the "proton-sponge effect" [112], and efficient escape of the nucleic acid cargo from endosomes.

One approach to enhance siRNA delivery with PEI is increasing the hydrophobicity of PEI by covalently conjugating alkyl chains [113], where increasing the hydrophobic alkyl chain length generally improved the stability of the PEI/siRNA complex. In a similar strategy, cholesterol was conjugated to PEI with decreased toxicity of the conjugates [114]. Low molecular weight PEI (MW < 5 kDa) is less toxic than the higher molecular weight PEI (≈25 kDa), but less efficient

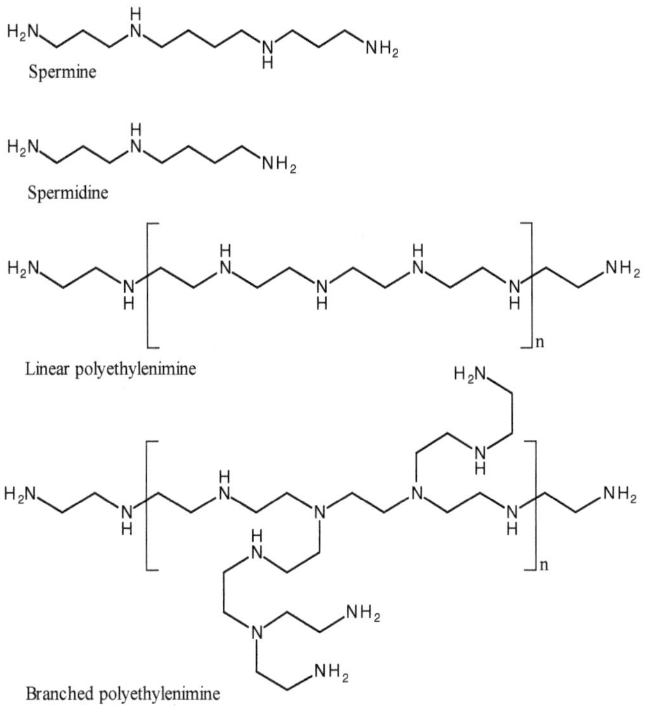

**Figure 6.** Representative examples of polyamines used in siRNA delivery either as in lipid conjugates of polyamine alkaloids e.g. spermine and spermidine, or as in polyethylenimine (PEI), a cationic polymer.

in polynucleotide delivery, thus, cross-linking of the low molecular weight PEI with disulfide bonds which are cleaved in the reducing environment of the cytoplasm increased the efficiency of siRNA delivery through the enhanced release of siRNA in the cytoplasm [115].

Chitosan is a biocompatible and biodegradable polysaccharide that is a copolymer of N-acetyl-D-glucosamine and D-glucosamine. Chitosan has weakly basic properties due to the presence of the D-glucosamine residue with a pKa value 6.2-7.0. The molecular weight of chitosan affects the complex stability, size, zeta-potential and in vitro gene knock-down of siRNA/chitosan nanoparticles [116]. High molecular weight (64.8-170 kDa) chitosan formed stable complexes with siRNA and resulted in high gene knock-down efficiency in human lung carcinoma (H1299) cells, while low molecular weight (10 kDa) chitosan could not complex the siRNA into stable nanoparticles and showed almost no knock-down [117]. The method of association affects gene silencing efficiency, where chitosan-TPP/siRNA nanoparticles (siRNA entrapped inside the nanoparticles, and TPP is sodium tripolyphosphate and used as a polyanion to cross-link with the cationic chitosan groups by electrostatic interactions) showed high siRNA binding and better gene silencing in vitro compared to siRNA/chitosan particles prepared by simple complexation and adsorption of siRNA onto chitosan [118]. Although chitosan has good potential as a non-viral gene delivery vector, widespread use is largely limited by its poor solubility (because of their pKa, chitosan amino groups are only partially protonated at the physiological pH 7.4), poor stability of its siRNA complexes at the physiological pH, and low transfection efficiency. Various strategies have been adopted to overcome these drawbacks, such as covalently conjugating PEG to chitosan and binding targeting ligands to enhance cell specificity [116].

Cyclodextrins (CD) are cyclic oligosaccharides composed of 6, 7, or 8 D-(+)-glucose units, known as $\alpha$-CD, $\beta$-CD, $\gamma$-CD respectively, bound through $\alpha$-1,4-linkages. Polymers conjugated to $\beta$-CD lack immunogenicity and hence are attractive vectors for polynucleotide delivery. $\beta$-CD have a hydrophilic outer surface and a hydrophobic inner cavity which enable them to form inclusion complexes. Efficient cellular transfection of siRNA labelled with a fluorescent tag into human embryonic lung fibroblasts (MRC-5 cells) was observed by siRNA complexes with the $\beta$-CD guanidine derivatized bis-(guanidinium)-tetrakis-($\beta$-cyclodextrin) tetrapod (having four $\beta$-CD units) [119]. The ability of $\beta$-CD to form inclusion complexes was used to develop a siRNA delivery vector. $\beta$-CD was covalently bound to a polycationic segment (to electrostatically bind siRNA), while adamantane-PEG-transferrin (adamantane can fit in the $\beta$-CD cavity) formed an inclusion complex which can enhance the stability of siRNA nanoparticles in vivo [120]. This system was used to deliver siRNA silencing the *EWS-FLI1* gene thus inhibiting tumour growth in a murine model of metastatic Ewing's sarcoma. The first experimental siRNA therapeutic to provide targeted delivery in humans was reported by Davis and co-workers [121]. siRNA was formulated into a nanoparticle (CALAA-01), which consisted of a cyclodextrin-containing polymer that contains amidine and primary amine functional groups, a PEG for steric stabilization in the in vivo environment (via inclusion complexes of $\beta$-CD with adamantine-PEG conjugate), and human transferrin (Tf) as the targeting ligand to binds to the transferrin receptors that are over-expressed on cancer cells. The siRNA/nanoparticles components self-assembled in the pharmacy. CALAA-01 was administered intravenously to the first patient with a solid cancer in a phase I clinical trial (safety study) in May 2008 [121]. Tumour biopsies from patients' melanoma after treatment (phase I clinical trial) showed the presence of intracellular nanoparticles. Reductions in the levels of both the specific mRNA (M2 subunit of ribonucleotide reductase, RRM2) and the protein (RRM2) were found when compared to levels in pre-dosing tissues. These results demonstrated that siRNA nanoparticles administered systemically to a human patient can produce a specific gene knock-down via an RNAi mechanism of action [122]. A recent and novel approach to the synthesis of cationic or neutral PEGylated amphiphilic $\beta$-CD used copper-catalysed "click" chemistry to modify selectively the secondary 2-hydroxyl group of the $\beta$-CD. The 6-position of these $\beta$-CD conjugates was conjugated to a dodecane alkyl chain. Complexation of cationic $\beta$-CD alone with siRNA resulted in good silencing of the luciferase reporter gene in Caco2 cells in culture. Co-formulation of cationic $\beta$-CD with a PEGylated $\beta$-CD and siRNA resulted in lower surface charges and reduced aggregation. The transfection efficiency of the cationic $\beta$-CD vector was lowered by co-formulation with the PEGylated $\beta$-CD, although the siRNA binding was not affected and the surface charge of the complexes did not reach complete neutrality [123].

Dendrimers have a central core to which are connected several branched arms in a manner that can be symmetrical or asymmetrical. During the synthesis of dendrimers, arms (branches) are added to the core structure. Each addition is called a generation and increases the previous generation number by one. Due to their unique structure, dendrimers can have a planar, elliptical, or spherical shape depending on generation number. Among the most widely used dendrimers are polyamidoamine (PAMAM) and polypropylenimine (PPI) dendrimers [124]. Dendrimers which have positively charged cationic groups on their outer surface are commonly used for polynucleotide delivery. The transfection efficiency of dendrimers increases with increasing the charge density or generation number [125]. However, dendrimers with high generation number are generally more cytotoxic compared to dendrimers with low generation number [126]. Usually the inner space near the core is larger compared to outer space near the surface due to the lower density of molecules (less number of arms) near the core, which allow small molecules to be incorporated in the inner space. Owing to the relatively large molecular weight of polynucleotides, they are usually bound to the surface of cationic dendrimers and not in the inner space of the dendrimer. Generally, the toxicity of dendrimers is lower than that of PEI or poly-L-lysine (PLL) [127]. One advantage of dendrimers is that they have pH buffering capacity (proton-sponge effect), an important feature for endosomal escape and enhancing the release of polynucleotides [125, 128].

PPI dendrimers with high generation numbers (4 and 5) were more efficient in forming discrete nanoparticles with siRNA and in gene silencing in human lung cancer (A549) cells than lower generation dendrimers (2 and 3). Generation 5 PPI dendrimers were more toxic, probably due to the increased positive charge density per dendrimer, than generation 4 dendrimers [129]. Complex formation between PAMAM dendrimers with an ethylenediamine core and siRNA as a function of three variables has been reported [130]. The ionic strength of the medium (without or with 150 mM NaCl), the generation number (4, 5, 6 and 7) and the $N/P$ ratio (ratio of positively charged amine groups per negative phosphate) were varied. The size of the complexes depended on the ionic strength of the media, with the strong electrostatic interactions in medium without NaCl making siRNA/dendrimer complexes smaller than those obtained in 150 mM NaCl. Both the intracellular delivery and the silencing of EGFP expression in cell culture was dependent on complex size, with smaller complexes efficiently delivered, and resulting in the highest silencing of EGFP expression. siRNA complexed with generation 7 dendrimers resulted in the highest silencing of EGFP expression both in human brain tumour cell line T98G-EGFP (35%) and mouse macrophage cell line J-774-EGFP (45%) cells, in spite of having lower protection of siRNA against degradation with RNase A, showing the importance of formulation procedures on the efficiency of transfection [130].

# 4. Cationic lipids as non-viral vectors for siRNA and DNA delivery

## 4.1. Gene delivery by cationic lipids

Gene delivery (DNA transfection) with cationic lipids (Figure 7) dates back to 1987 when it was reported by Felgner et al. [131], and the term "lipofection" was coined. Small unilamellar liposomes containing the cationic lipid N-[1-(2,3-dioleyloxy)propyl]-N,N,N-trimethyl ammonium chloride (DOTMA) was reported to spontaneously complex DNA completely entrapping the DNA, and enhanced fusion with the cell membrane in vitro in cell cultures, resulting in efficient delivery and expression of the delivered DNA. The lipofection was 5-100-fold more effective than the commonly used transfection techniques at the time by either calcium phosphate or DEAE-dextran (diethylaminoethyl-dextran), depending on the cell line used [131]. Cationic lipids have polar and non-polar domains and thus are amphiphilic in nature, with three general structural domains: (a) a cationic hydrophilic head-group (positively charged). The head-group can carry a permanent positive charge as in quaternary ammonium groups, or can be protonated at the physiological pH 7.4, such as primary and secondary amine groups. There can be one cationic group per lipid molecule (monovalent cationic lipids) or more than one cationic group per lipid molecule (multivalent cationic lipids); (b) a hydrophobic domain covalently attached by a linker to the cationic head-group. This domain can be in the form of either alkyl chains (commonly 2 chains) of various chain lengths (with various oxidation states) or can be a steroid such as cholesterol; (c) the linker between the head-group and the hydrophobic domain [132, 133]. This linker controls the biodegradation of the cationic lipid and its stability under different conditions according to the type of chemical bonds (e.g. ester, ether, or amide). Each domain can be controlled to change a specific character of the cationic lipid, e.g. using a disulfide functional group as a bioresponsive linker [134] which is reduced in the intracellular environment by glutathione/glutathione reductase and enhance biodegradation characters of the lipid and decrease its cytotoxicity.

## 4.2. The cationic head-group

The cationic head-group's main function is to bind electrostatically the negatively charged phosphates of the polynucleotides. The complexes of cationic lipids with polynucleotides such as DNA and siRNA are called lipoplexes. This requires the presence of a positive charge on the head-group at the physiological pH 7.4, i.e. the pKa of the head-group is ideally at least one unit higher than the physiological pH. The most commonly used head-groups contain nitrogen (e.g. amines or guanidines). However other head-groups, e.g. arsonium and phosphonium have been reported [135]. Arsonium is less toxic than arsenic (III), and in vitro cytotoxicity evaluation showed that arsonium and phosphonium are surprisingly less toxic than the ammonium group [135, 136].

One property that can be changed by controlling the type of the head-group is the head-group cross-sectional area. The greater the difference between the cross-sectional area of the polar head-group and that of the hydrophobic domain, when the former is designed to be smaller than the latter, the greater is the ability of the cationic lipid to fuse with the cell membrane and endosomal membrane and the greater is the release of polynucleotides from their complex with the cationic lipid due to the decreased structural stability of the lipid assembly [133, 137]. The hydration of the head-group affects its cross-sectional area, thus, the conjugation of groups which decrease the hydration state (such as hydroxyalkyl groups that form intermolecular H-bonds) decreases the head-group cross-sectional area.

Thus, gene delivery by DOTMA and DOTAP (1,2-dioleoyloxy-3-(trimethylammonio)-propane) was enhanced by incorporation of a hydroxyethyl group to yield the lipids DORIE

(1,2-dioleyloxypropyl-3-dimethyl-hydroxyethyl ammonium bromide) and DORI (N-[1-(2,3-dioleoyloxy)propyl-N-[1-(2-hydroxy)ethyl]-N,N-dimethyl ammonium iodide) respectively [138, 139]. The head-group cross-sectional area can be also controlled by subtle changes to the head-group structure. The DC-Chol (3β(N-(N',N'-dimethylaminoethane)carbamoyl)cholesterol) with dimethylamino head-group resulted in more efficient transfection compared to DC-Chol with diethylamino or diisopropylamino head-groups, probably due to increased steric repulsion of the head-groups.

The in vitro gene transfer with six non-cholesterol-based cationic lipids (each having two alkyl chains) with a single guanidinium head-group in Chinese hamster ovary (CHO), COS-1, MCF-7, A549, and HepG2 cells has been reported [140]. These lipids were able to form lipoplexes with size-range 200-600 nm and ζ-potential +3.4 to -34 mV. The efficiencies of the lipids which had an extra quaternized cationic centre were 2-4-fold more than that of the commercially available reagent Lipofectamine in transfecting COS-1, CHO, A-549, and MCF-7 cells. MTT viability assay in CHO cells showed high (>75%) cell viabilities at the lipid/DNA charge ratios used. DNase I protection assays showed that the lipids having the extra quaternized centre protected DNA better against enzyme catalysed hydrolysis. These results shed light on the importance of choosing the type of head-group and number of cationic centres in designing cationic lipids [140].

A series of cationic cholesterol derivatives were synthesized by covalently attaching the heterocycles imidazole, piperazine, pyridine, and morpholine groups (the head-groups) to the parent cholesterol via a biodegradable carbamoyl linker [141]. These lipids were compared with the parent DC-Chol with the linear amine head-group, and they generally showed better or comparable transfection efficiency of pCMV-luciferase into human HepG2 cells (a human liver cancer cell line) in the presence or absence of FCS. The most efficient two of these lipids were with morpholine and piperazine head-groups, and they gave higher levels of gene expression in HepG2 and human melanoma cell line (KZ2) which are generally very hard to transfect with the commonly used reagents e.g. DC-Chol, Lipofectamine, and PEI. In vivo studies with lipids having morpholine and piperazine head-groups resulted in successful delivery of the reporter gene to the target cells through intrasplenic injection [141]. Cationic lipids which have more than one cationic head-group (multivalent cationic lipids) have more surface charge density than their monovalent (with one head-group) analogues, and they are generally expected to better bind and complex polynucleotides. Many multivalent cationic lipids contain a natural occurring polyamine such as spermidine and spermine, which are believed to interact with the minor groove of B-DNA [142].

The triamine spermidine and the tetramine spermine (Figure 6), and their diamine precursor putrescine, are organic polycations that are widely but unevenly distributed in both mammalian and non-mammalian cells and tissues. They have an essential role in controlling DNA, RNA and protein synthesis during normal and neoplastic growth, in cell differentiation, and tissue regeneration [143]. These polyamines exhibit many metabolic and neurophysiological effects in the nervous system, and are important for the developing and mature nervous system and affect modulation of ionic channels and calcium-dependent transmitter release [143-149].

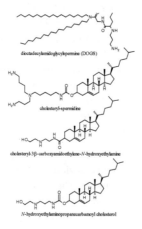

N-[1-(2,3-dioleyloxy)propyl]-N,N,N-trimethylammonium chloride (DOTMA)

1,2-dioleoyloxy-3-(trimethylammonio)-propane chloride (DOTAP)

3β(N-(N',N'-dimethylaminoethane)carbamoyl)-cholesterol hydrochloride (DC-Chol)

N-[1-(2,3-dioleoyloxy)propyl-N-[1-(2-hydroxy)ethyl]-N,N-dimethylammonium iodide (DORI)

1,2-dioleyloxypropyl-3-dimethyl-hydroxyethylammonium bromide (DORIE)

1,2-dimyristyloxypropyl-3-dimethyl-hydroxyethylammonium bromide (DMRIE)

dioctadecylamidoglycylspermine (DOGS)

cholesteryl-spermidine

cholesteryl-3β-carboxyamidoethylene-N-hydroxyethylamine

N-hydroxyethylaminopropanecarbamoyl cholesterol

**Figure 7.** Representative examples of cationic lipids used in DNA and siRNA delivery.

Spermine is incorporated in the cationic polymer polyspermine imidazole-4,5-imine (PSI) and in dioctadecylamidoglycyl-spermine (DOGS) [150] (Figure 7); spermidine is bound in cholesteryl-spermidine [151]. The free amine groups of spermine in cholesteryl-spermine conjugates have different p$K$a values and provide a buffering effect in the endosomes facilitating the escape of lipoplex from the endosomes [152]. The length of the linear polyamine attached to the hydrophobic domain and the charge distribution on it affects the transfection efficiency of the cationic lipid [153]. Addition of amine groups separated by methylene groups to the linear polyamine attached to a cholesterol residue did not automatically increase transfection efficiency regardless of the increased charge density. Molecular modelling simulations suggested that increasing chain length led to an increased number of folded conformations due to greater flexibility of the conjugates, which is unfavourable for interaction with DNA [132, 153].

The central tetramethylene motif of spermine was reported to be essential in conferring high transfection efficiency in a series of cholesterol-polyamine conjugates [152]. It was suggested that the tetramethylene segment of spermine can bridge between the DNA complementary strands, while the polyamine with a central trimethylene segment would only bind with the adjacent phosphates on the same DNA strand. These results point to the importance of the structure of the polyamine head-group and the relation between its amine groups, and also point to the fact that increasing efficiency of transfection is not only a matter of increasing the number of positive charges per head-group.

### 4.3. The hydrophobic domain

The length, saturation state and type of the hydrophobic chains conjugated to cationic lipids affect their transfection efficiency [154-156]. Although these factors were studied extensively for the effect on transfection, and although the majority of studies accepted that the type of alkyl chains influence the outcome of transfection, it is difficult to set a definitive set of rules to describe the best type of alkyl chains to be conjugated to the polar head-groups. The contribution of the alkyl chains (and the hydrophobic domain) to the cationic lipid properties as a whole is what determines the transfection efficiency of the lipid.

Results obtained with DMRIE (1,2-dimyristyloxypropyl-3-dimethylhydroxyethyl-ammonium bromide) [157], glycine betaine conjugates [138] with two alkyl chains, alkyl acyl carnitine esters having chains of length C12 to C18 [158], lactic acid conjugates of $N,N$-dialkyl amine group [159], lipids related to DOTAP with two alkyl chains (C12-C18) linked to the head-group through ether bonds [160], and cationic lipids with different hydroxyethyl or dihydroxypropyl ammonium backbones and esterified hydrocarbon chains and hydroxyl substituents [161] showed that a comparison of the cationic lipids based only on the lengths of the two saturated aliphatic chains led to the observation of the superior transfection efficiency of C14 chains over the longer C16 and C18 chains [132, 133]. It was proposed that a shorter chain length facilitates mixing with cellular membranes [138] which is important for endosomal escape [162].

In another set of experiments, we showed the longer chain C18 oleoyl (with one *cis*-double bond) to be more efficient than cationic lipids with shorter chain lengths. Varying the chain length in $N^4,N^9$-diacyl spermines from C10 to C18, for plasmid DNA delivery, resulted in us establishing that the conjugate with C18 oleoyl chains is both more efficient and less toxic than the shorter chain conjugates [163]. A series of multivalent Gemini-surfactants with the hydrophobic chains systematically varied resulted in the conjugates with C18 oleoyl chains to be better in transfection than the C16 and C14 alkyl chains [164]. Chain saturation was also shown to affect the efficiency of transfection. The results of studies on a set of cationic triester phosphatidyl choline derivatives (each having two alkyl chains) show a strong dependence of their transfection efficiency on the lipid hydrocarbon chain characteristics, where transfection activity increases with increasing chain unsaturation from fully saturated to having two double bonds. Transfection efficiency decreased with increasing chain length (increasing the total number of carbons per lipid molecule ~30-50). Maximum transfection was with monounsaturated myristoleoyl 14:1 chains [156]. The data obtained from transfection experiments with 20 cationic phosphatidylcholine (PC) derivatives show that hydrocarbon chain variations results in transfection efficiencies that varies by more than 2 orders of magnitude. The most important variables were chain saturation state and total number of carbon atoms in the lipid chains. Transfection increased with decreasing chain length and increasing chain unsaturation. Best transfection efficiency was found for cationic lipids with monounsaturated (myristoleoyl) 14:1 chains [154]. Higher levels of transfection were also reported with lipids having oleoyl chains in comparison with stearoyl chains [157, 158]. Unsaturated chains promote lipid fusion between the lipoplexes and the various cellular membranes, which is essential for delivery and endosomal escape [133, 154, 165].

Cholesterol derivatives with various cationic head-groups were synthesized to investigate their efficiency as siRNA delivery vectors. The transfection efficiencies of siRNA lipoplexes prepared with the cationic cholesterol derivatives DC-Chol, cholesteryl-3β-carboxyamido-ethylene-N-hydroxyethylamine (OH-Chol), and N-hydroxyethylaminopropane carbamoyl cholesterol (HAPC) was investigated in human prostate tumour cells that stably express the luciferase gene (PC-3-Luc). When lipoplexes were prepared in water, HAPC was more effective in knocking-down luciferase activity than OH-Chol and DC-Chol [166]. The presence of NaCl while preparing the lipoplexes increased the gene silencing efficiency of luciferase, while it did not affect efficiency of HAPC. The commercially available transfection reagent, Lipofectamine 2000 (a cationic lipid liposomal preparation) resulted in strong gene silencing by siRNA, but exhibited increased toxicity (~40% cell viability), in contrast to OH-Chol, DC-Chol, and HAPC lipoplexes (~80–100% cell viability). These results indicated that siRNA lipoplexes prepared with OH-Chol, and HAPC can efficiently suppress gene expression without increased cytotoxicity [166].

## 4.4. The linker

The linker is dependent upon the type (hence properties) of the functional group and its length (number of carbon atoms). The linker has two main functions: (a) to conjugate covalently the polar head-group to the hydrophobic domain; (b) to control the biodegradability of the cationic lipid and/or introduce a new property to the cationic lipid, e.g. responding to the intracellular reducing environment [133, 167]. The most commonly used linker functional groups are: amide, carbamate, ester, ether, ortho ester, and disulfide.

Both amides and ester bonds are biodegradable and hence are hypothesized to be less toxic than other non-biodegradable bonds (e.g. ethers) [168]. Lipids with a pyridinium head-group (with palmitoyl 16:0 hydrophobic domains and with ester and amide linkers) were used to prepare liposomes with either DOPE or cholesterol at the cationic lipid/helper-lipid molar ratio of 1:1. Following transfection of CHO cells with lipoplexes delivering plasmids expressing EGFP, the cationic lipids having amide linkers significantly increased transfection efficiency in all liposomal formulations compared to their counterparts having the ester linker [169]. The high transfection efficiency of lipids with amide linker was suggested to be due to their lower phase-transition temperature which makes the liposome's bilayer structure more stable in aqueous media during the transfection process as well as liposome storage. The phase-transition temperature of a lipid is the temperature at which there is a change in the lipid's physical state from the ordered gel phase (where the hydrocarbon chains are closely packed and fully extended) to the disordered liquid crystalline phase (where the hydrocarbon chains are fluid and randomly orientated) [169].

Depending on the structure of the cationic lipid, the linker influence on transfection efficiency can be more than on cytotoxicity. Cholesterol-based cationic lipids that have different nitro-genous heterocyclic head-groups (N-methylimidazole, N-methylmorpholine, and pyridine) and acid-labile linkers (carbamate, ester, and N,O-acetal ether) were used to transfect human embryonic kidney 293 (HEK 293) cells with EGFP plasmid [170]. Choosing those linkers was based on the concept that incorporation of acid-labile bonds in the cationic lipid structure enhances the release of polynucleotides from the endosomes, therefore increasing the trans-fection efficiency [171]. N,O-Acetals are known to undergo hydrolysis in acidic environment [170, 171]. The results showed that the structure of these lipids only slightly affected their cytotoxicity but largely changes the efficiency of intracellular accumulation of the polynu-cleotides. The lipids having the cationic head-groups pyridine and/or methylimidazole head-groups with either an ester or a carbamate linker resulted in better transfection efficiency as compared with the cationic lipids with either the N-methylmorpholine head-groups and/or an ether linker. The lipid that has a pyridine head-group and a carbamate linker to deliver EGFP plasmid resulted in comparable transfection efficiency with that achieved with com-mercially available Lipofectamine 2000.

Two cleavable cationic lipids having a linear or a cyclic ortho-ester linker between the cationic head-group and the unsaturated hydrophobic domain (two oleoyl chains) were previously reported [172]. It is hypothesized that the acidic pH in the endosomes catalyzes the hydrolysis of the linker group to result in fragmentation products that destabilize the endosomal mem-branes. At pH 7.4, the lipids (with DOPE) formed stable lipoplexes with plasmid DNA. Decreas-ing the pH enhanced the hydrolysis of the ortho ester linkers which removed the cationic head-groups and caused lipoplex aggregation. At pH 5.5, the cationic lipid N-[2-methyl-2-(1',2'-dioleylglyceroxy)dioxolan-4-yl]methyl-N,N,N-trimethylammonium iodide that have a cyclic ortho-ester linker showed increased pH-sensitivity and caused the permeation of its lipoplexes to model biomembranes within the time span of endosomal processing before the lysosomal degradation. This lipid markedly increased gene transfection (~3-50-fold) of the luciferase reporter protein in monkey kidney fibroblast (CV-1) and human breast cancer (HTB-129) cells in culture compared to the pH-insensitive control lipid DOTAP lipoplexes [172].

Transfection with DNA lipoplexes of three thiocholesterol-derived gemini cationic lipids possessing disulfide linkages incorporated between the cationic head-group and the thiocholesterol backbone in order to render the lipids biodegradable has been reported [173]. Comparing transfection in a prostate cancer line (PC3AR) and a human keratinocyte cell line (HaCat) with two commercially available reagents showed comparable or better expression of GFP in the transfected cells. Cytotoxicity studies showed the nontoxic property of these lipid-DNA complexes at different $N/P$ ratios used for transfection studies. The rationale behind this design was to ensure the destabilization of the lipid-polynucleotide lipoplexes in the cytoplasm after reduction of the disulfide linker by the intracellular glutathione (GSH), which is the most abundant low molecular weight thiol present in cells and is involved in controlling cellular redox environment. GSH is found at very high intracellular concentrations and at comparatively low extracellular concentrations e.g. blood plasma concentrations (2 µM) are 1000-fold less than concentration in erythrocytes (2 mM). This large difference between intra- and extracellular environments provides a potential mechanism for release of polynucleotides from lipoplexes of lipids that have a disulfide functional group linker and is now a well-trodden research path [115, 134, 173].

## 5. Conclusions and future avenues

In our research, symmetrical and asymmetrical acyl polyamine derivatives (fatty acid amides of spermine) [152] have been synthesized, characterized, and evaluated as non-viral vectors for siRNA [163, 174-177]. The intracellular delivery of siRNA and the subsequent sequence specific gene silencing has been quantified by flow cytometry techniques (FACS analysis) [163]. The ability of the spermine conjugates to bind siRNA and form nanoparticles has been investigated and the effect of the complexes of siRNA lipoplexes on the cell viability 48 h post-transfection has been quantified. Our SAR studies allow the identification of the most efficient fatty acids in terms of high gene-silencing efficiency and high cell viability [174-178].

Whilst we were completing this Chapter, four interesting papers, each one on a different aspect of this topic, were published. Langer, Anderson and co-workers at MIT reported on the delivery of immunostimulatory RNA (isRNA) to Toll-like receptor (TLR)-expressing cells to drive innate and adaptive immune responses. The specific activation of TLRs has potential for a variety of therapeutic indications including antiviral immunotherapy and as vaccine adjuvants. Effective lipidoid-isRNA nanoparticles, when tested in mice, stimulated strong IFN-α responses following subcutaneous injection, had robust antiviral activity that suppressed influenza virus replication, and enhanced antiovalbumin humoral and cell-mediated responses when used as a vaccine adjuvant. Their lipidoid formulations, designed specifically for the delivery of isRNA to TLRs, were superior to the commonly used N-[1-(2,3-dioleoyloxy)propyl]-N,N,N-trimethylammonium methylsulfate-RNA delivery system and may provide new tools for the manipulation of TLR responses in vitro and in vivo [179]. This paper follows after their other recent major contribution on delivering naked siRNA as part of a self-assembled (due to DNA complementarity) tetrahedral nanoparticle construct considering the presentation of folate as a cancer targeting ligand [180]. These monodisperse nanoparticles of essentially naked DNA, carrying siRNA as the cargo, have a defined size of only a few nm. They show that at least three folate molecules per nanoparticle are required for optimal delivery of the siRNA into cells and that gene silencing only occurs when the ligands are appropriately orientated. In vivo, these naked DNA nanoparticles showed a longer blood circulation time than the parent siRNA [180]. In another exciting development, Geall and co-workers at Novartis have also advanced the field of nucleic acid vaccines by taking advantage of the recent innovations in non-viral systemic delivery of siRNA using lipid nanoparticles (LNPs) to develop a self-amplifying RNA vaccine. This technology elicited broad, potent, and protective immune responses, comparable with those achieved by a viral delivery system, but without the inherent limitations of viral vectors [181]. Even today, a biologically responsive cationic polymer system based on spermine has been reported for the intracellular delivery of siRNA [182]. This polyspermine imidazole-4,5-imine (PSI) (Figure 7) carrier is designed to be hydrolysed at the mildly acidic pH found in the endosome.

It is clear that both ssRNA to activate the immune system and RNAi brought about by siRNA delivery have high therapeutic potential. The major remaining barrier, that of efficient and potentially selective delivery to target cells in now being addressed. The non-viral delivery of siRNA is a major tool in modern functional genomics. Medicines design, the formulation of drugs, in this case siRNA and plasmid DNA, is an essential requirement for efficient gene therapy.

## Acknowledgements

We thank the Egyptian Government for a fully-funded studentship to AAM.

## Author details

Ian S. Blagbrough[1] and Abdelkader A. Metwally[1,2]

*Address all correspondence to: prsisb@bath.ac.uk

1 Department of Pharmacy and Pharmacology, University of Bath, Bath BA2 7AY, UK

2 Department of Pharmaceutics and Industrial Pharmacy, Faculty of Pharmacy, Ain Shams University, Abbasya, Cairo, Egypt

## References

[1] Blagbrough IS, Zara C. Animal Models for Target Diseases in Gene Therapy - Using DNA and siRNA Delivery Strategies. Pharmaceutical Research 2009;26(1) 1-18.

[2]  van der Krol AR, Mur LA, Beld M, Mol J, Stuitje AR. Flavonoid Genes in Petunia: Addition of a Limited Number of Gene Copies May Lead to a Suppression of Gene Expression. The Plant Cell Online 1990;2(4) 291-299.

[3]  Napoli C, Lemieux C, Jorgensen R. Introduction of a Chimeric Chalcone Synthase Gene into Petunia Results in Reversible Co-Suppression of Homologous Genes *in Trans*. The Plant Cell Online 1990;2(4) 279-289.

[4]  Vanblokland R, Vandergeest N, Mol JNM, Kooter JM. Transgene-Mediated Suppression of Chalcone Synthase Expression in Petunia Hybrida Results from an Increase in RNA Turnover. Plant Journal 1994;6(6) 861-877.

[5]  Metzlaff M, Odell M, Cluster PD, Flavell RB. RNA-Mediated RNA Degradation and Chalcone Synthase a Silencing in Petunia. Cell 1997;88(6) 845-854.

[6]  Hamilton AJ, Baulcombe DC. A Species of Small Antisense RNA in Posttranscriptional Gene Silencing in Plants. Science 1999;286(5441) 950-952. DOI: 10.1126/science. 286.5441.950.

[7]  Hamilton A, Voinnet O, Chappell L, Baulcombe D. Two Classes of Short Interfering RNA in RNA Silencing. EMBO Journal 2002;21(17) 4671-4679. DOI: 10.1093/emboj/cdf464.

[8]  Baumberger N, Baulcombe DC. Arabidopsis Argonaute1 Is an RNA Slicer That Selectively Recruits microRNAs and Short Interfering RNAs. Proceedings of the National Academy of Sciences of the United States of America 2005;102(33) 11928-11933. DOI: 10.1073/pnas.0505461102.

[9]  Fire A, Xu SQ, Montgomery MK, Kostas SA, Driver SE, Mello CC. Potent and Specific Genetic Interference by Double-Stranded RNA in Caenorhabditis Elegans. Nature 1998;391(6669) 806-811.

[10]  Elbashir SM, Harborth J, Lendeckel W, Yalcin A, Weber K, Tuschl T. Duplexes of 21-Nucleotide RNAs Mediate RNA Interference in Cultured Mammalian Cells. Nature 2001;411(6836) 494-498.

[11]  Skloot R. The Immortal Life of Henrietta Lacks. London, UK: Macmillan; 2010.

[12]  Cogoni C, Macino G. Post-Transcriptional Gene Silencing across Kingdoms. Current Opinion in Genetics and Development 2000;10(6) 638-643.

[13]  Sontheimer EJ. Assembly and Function of RNA Silencing Complexes. Nature Reviews Molecular Cell Biology 2005;6(2) 127-138.

[14]  Collins RE, Cheng XD. Structural and Biochemical Advances in Mammalian RNAi. Journal of Cellular Biochemistry 2006;99(5) 1251-1266.

[15]  Hutvagner G, Simard MJ. Argonaute Proteins: Key Players in RNA Silencing. Nature Reviews Molecular Cell Biology 2008;9(1) 22-32.

[16] Gaynor JW, Campbell BJ, Cosstick R. RNA Interference: A Chemist's Perspective. Chemical Society Reviews 2010;39(11) 4169-4184.

[17] Liu QH, Paroo Z. Biochemical Principles of Small RNA Pathways. Annual Review of Biochemistry 2010;79 295-319.

[18] Haley B, Zamore PD. Kinetic Analysis of the RNAi Enzyme Complex. Nature Structural & Molecular Biology 2004;11(7) 599-606.

[19] Hutvagner G. Small RNA Asymmetry in RNAi: Function in Risc Assembly and Gene Regulation. FEBS Letters 2005;579(26) 5850-5857.

[20] Wang HW, Noland C, Siridechadilok B, Taylor DW, Ma EB, Felderer K, Doudna JA, Nogales E. Structural Insights into RNA Processing by the Human Risc-Loading Complex. Nature Structural & Molecular Biology 2009;16(11) 1148-1153.

[21] Wahid F, Shehzad A, Khan T, Kim YY. MicroRNAs: Synthesis, Mechanism, Function, and Recent Clinical Trials. Biochimica et Biophysica Acta (BBA) - Molecular Cell Research 2010;1803(11) 1231-1243.

[22] Paddison PJ, Caudy AA, Bernstein E, Hannon GJ, Conklin DS. Short Hairpin RNAs (shRNAs) Induce Sequence-Specific Silencing in Mammalian Cells. Genes & Development 2002;16(8) 948-958.

[23] Rao DD, Vorhies JS, Senzer N, Nemunaitis J. siRNA Vs. shRNA: Similarities and Differences. Advanced Drug Delivery Reviews 2009;61(9) 746-759.

[24] Freier SM, Kierzek R, Jaeger JA, Sugimoto N, Caruthers MH, Neilson T, Turner DH. Improved Free-Energy Parameters for Predictions of RNA Duplex Stability. Proceedings of the National Academy of Sciences of the United States of America 1986;83(24) 9373-9377.

[25] Freier SM, Altmann KH. The Ups and Downs of Nucleic Acid Duplex Stability: Structure-Stability Studies on Chemically-Modified DNA:RNA Duplexes. Nucleic Acids Research 1997;25(22) 4429-4443.

[26] Beverly MB. Applications of Mass Spectrometry to the Study of siRNA. Mass Spectrometry Reviews 2010; 10.1002/mas.20260.

[27] Shah SA, Brunger AT. The 1.8 Angstrom Crystal Structure of a Statically Disordered 17 Base-Pair RNA Duplex: Principles of RNA Crystal Packing and Its Effect on Nucleic Acid Structure. Journal of Molecular Biology 1999;285(4) 1577-1588.

[28] Rana TM. Illuminating the Silence: Understanding the Structure and Function of Small RNAs. Nature Reviews Molecular Cell Biology 2007;8(1) 23-36.

[29] Banan M, Puri N. The Ins and Outs of RNAi in Mammalian Cells. Current Pharmaceutical Biotechnology 2004;5(5) 441-450.

[30]  Hickerson RP, Vlassov AV, Wang Q, Leake D, Ilves H, Gonzalez-Gonzalez E, Contag CH, Johnston BH, Kaspar RL. Stability Study of Unmodified siRNA and Relevance to Clinical Use. Oligonucleotides 2008;18(4) 345-354.

[31]  Layzer JM, McCaffrey AP, Tanner AK, Huang Z, Kay MA, Sullenger BA. In Vivo Activity of Nuclease-Resistant siRNA. RNA-a Publication of the Rna Society 2004;10(5) 766-771.

[32]  Turner JJ, Jones SW, Moschos SA, Lindsay MA, Gait MJ. Maldi-Tof Mass Spectral Analysis of siRNA Degradation in Serum Confirms an RNase a-Like Activity. Molecular Biosystems 2007;3(1) 43-50.

[33]  Volkov AA, Kruglova NyS, Meschaninova MI, Venyaminova AG, Zenkova MA, Vlassov VV, Chernolovskaya EL. Selective Protection of Nuclease-Sensitive Sites in siRNA Prolongs Silencing Effect. Oligonucleotides 2009;19(2) 191-202.

[34]  Melnikova I. RNA-Based Therapies. Nature Reviews Drug Discovery 2007;6(11) 863-864.

[35]  Skoblov M. Prospects of Antisense Therapy Technologies. Molecular Biology 2009;43(6) 917-929.

[36]  Ghosal A, Kabir AH, Mandal A. RNA Interference and Its Therapeutic Potential. Central European Journal of Medicine 2011;6(2) 137-147.

[37]  Cheng H, Luo C, Wu X, Zhang Y, He Y, Wu Q, Xia Y, Zhang J. shRNA Targeting Plcε Inhibits Bladder Cancer Growth in Vitro and in Vivo. Urology 2011;78(2).

[38]  Qin X-J, Dai D-J, Gao Z-G, Huan J-L, Zhu L. Effect of Lentivirus-Mediated shRNA Targeting Vegfr-3 on Proliferation, Apoptosis and Invasion of Gastric Cancer Cells. International Journal of Molecular Medicine 2011;28(5) 761-768.

[39]  Liu Q-S, Zhang J, Liu M, Dong W-G. Lentiviral-Mediated miRNA against Liver-Intestine Cadherin Suppresses Tumor Growth and Invasiveness of Human Gastric Cancer. Cancer Science 2010;101(8) 1807-1812.

[40]  Bumcrot D, Manoharan M, Koteliansky V, Sah DWY. RNAi Therapeutics: A Potential New Class of Pharmaceutical Drugs. Nature Chemical Biology 2006;2(12) 711-719.

[41]  Aleku M, Schulz P, Keil O, Santel A, Schaeper U, Dieckhoff B, Janke O, Endruschat J, Durieux B, Roeder N, Loeffler K, Lange C, Fechtner M, Moepert K, Fisch G, Dames S, Arnold W, Jochims K, Giese K, Wiedenmann B, Scholz A, Kaufmann J. Atu027, a Liposomal Small Interfering RNA Formulation Targeting Protein Kinase N3, Inhibits Cancer Progression. Cancer Research 2008;68(23) 9788-9798.

[42]  Behlke MA. Progress Towards in Vivo Use of siRNA. Molecular Therapy 2006;13(4) 644-670.

[43]  Whitehead KA, Langer R, Anderson DG. Knocking Down Barriers: Advances in siRNA Delivery. Nature Reviews Drug Discovery 2009;8(2) 129-138.

[44] Reischl D, Zimmer A. Drug Delivery of siRNA Therapeutics: Potentials and Limits of Nanosystems. Nanomedicine: Nanotechnology, Biology and Medicine 2009;5(1) 8-20.

[45] van de Water FM, Boerman OC, Wouterse AC, Peters JGP, Russel FGM, Masereeuw R. Intravenously Administered Short Interfering RNA Accumulates in the Kidney and Selectively Suppresses Gene Function in Renal Proximal Tubules. Drug Metabolism and Disposition 2006;34(8) 1393-1397.

[46] Ruponen M, Ronkko S, Honkakoski P, Pelkonen J, Tammi M, Urtti A. Extracellular Glycosaminoglycans Modify Cellular Trafficking of Lipoplexes and Polyplexes. Journal of Biological Chemistry 2001;276(36) 33875-33880.

[47] Singh AK, Kasinath BS, Lewis EJ. Interaction of Polycations with Cell-Surface Negative Charges of Epithelial-Cells. Biochimica et Biophysica Acta 1992;1120(3) 337-342.

[48] Watts JK, Deleavey GF, Damha MJ. Chemically Modified siRNA: Tools and Applications. Drug Discovery Today 2008;13(19-20) 842-855.

[49] Behlke MA. Chemical Modification of siRNAs for in Vivo Use. Oligonucleotides 2008;18(4) 305-319.

[50] Hall AHS, Wan J, Shaughnessy EE, Shaw BR, Alexander KA. RNA Interference Using Boranophosphate siRNAs: Structure-Activity Relationships. Nucleic Acids Research 2004;32(20) 5991-6000.

[51] Ui-Tei K, Naito Y, Zenno S, Nishi K, Yamato K, Takahashi F, Juni A, Saigo K. Functional Dissection of siRNA Sequence by Systematic DNA Substitution: Modified siRNA with a DNA Seed Arm Is a Powerful Tool for Mammalian Gene Silencing with Significantly Reduced Off-Target Effect. Nucleic Acids Research 2008;36(7) 2136-2151.

[52] Chiu YL, Rana TM. siRNA Function in RNAi: A Chemical Modification Analysis. RNA-a Publication of the Rna Society 2003;9(9) 1034-1048.

[53] Bell NM, Micklefield J. Chemical Modification of Oligonucleotides for Therapeutic, Bioanalytical and Other Applications. ChemBioChem 2009;10(17) 2691-2703.

[54] Corey DR. Chemical Modification: The Key to Clinical Application of RNA Interference? Journal of Clinical Investigation 2007;117(12) 3615-3622.

[55] Nishina K, Unno T, Uno Y, Kubodera T, Kanouchi T, Mizusawa H, Yokota T. Efficient in Vivo Delivery of siRNA to the Liver by Conjugation of Alpha-Tocopherol. Molecular Therapy 2008;16(4) 734-740.

[56] Lorenz C, Hadwiger P, John M, Vornlocher HP, Unverzagt C. Steroid and Lipid Conjugates of siRNAs to Enhance Cellular Uptake and Gene Silencing in Liver Cells. Bioorganic & Medicinal Chemistry Letters 2004;14(19) 4975-4977.

[57] Soutschek J, Akinc A, Bramlage B, Charisse K, Constien R, Donoghue M, Elbashir S, Geick A, Hadwiger P, Harborth J, John M, Kesavan V, Lavine G, Pandey RK, Racie T,

Rajeev KG, Rohl I, Toudjarska I, Wang G, Wuschko S, Bumcrot D, Koteliansky V, Limmer S, Manoharan M, Vornlocher HP. Therapeutic Silencing of an Endogenous Gene by Systemic Administration of Modified siRNAs. Nature 2004;432(7014) 173-178.

[58] Wolfrum C, Shi S, Jayaprakash KN, Jayaraman M, Wang G, Pandey RK, Rajeev KG, Nakayama T, Charrise K, Ndungo EM, Zimmermann T, Koteliansky V, Manoharan M, Stoffel M. Mechanisms and Optimization of in Vivo Delivery of Lipophilic siR-NAs. Nature Biotechnology 2007;25(10) 1149-1157.

[59] Eguchi A, Dowdy SF. siRNA Delivery Using Peptide Transduction Domains. Trends in Pharmacological Sciences 2009;30(7) 341-345.

[60] Muratovska A, Eccles MR. Conjugate for Efficient Delivery of Short Interfering RNA (siRNA) into Mammalian Cells. FEBS Letters 2004;558(1-3) 63-68.

[61] Moschos SA, Jones SW, Perry MM, Williams AE, Erjefalt JS, Turner JJ, Barnes PJ, Sproat BS, Gait MJ, Lindsay MA. Lung Delivery Studies Using siRNA Conjugated to Tat(48-60) and Penetratin Reveal Peptide Induced Reduction in Gene Expression and Induction of Innate Immunity. Bioconjugate Chemistry 2007;18(5) 1450-1459.

[62] Kim SH, Jeong JH, Lee SH, Kim SW, Park TG. Peg Conjugated Vegf siRNA for Anti-Angiogenic Gene Therapy. Journal of Controlled Release 2006;116(2) 123-129.

[63] Xia CF, Zhang Y, Boado RJ, Pardridge WM. Intravenous siRNA of Brain Cancer with Receptor Targeting and Avidin-Biotin Technology. Pharmaceutical Research 2007;24(12) 2309-2316.

[64] Chu TC, Twu KY, Ellington AD, Levy M. Aptamer Mediated siRNA Delivery. Nucleic Acids Research 2006;34(10).

[65] Li MJ, Bauer G, Michienzi A, Yee JK, Lee NS, Kim J, Li S, Castanotto D, Zaia J, Rossi JJ. Inhibition of HIV-1 Infection by Lentiviral Vectors Expressing Pol Iii-Promoted Anti-HIV RNAs. Molecular Therapy 2003;8(2) 196-206.

[66] Sliva K, Schnierle BS. Selective Gene Silencing by Viral Delivery of Short Hairpin RNA. Virology Journal 2010;7 248.

[67] Berkowitz R, Ilves H, Lin WY, Eckert K, Coward A, Tamaki S, Veres G, Plavec I. Construction and Molecular Analysis of Gene Transfer Systems Derived from Bovine Immunodeficiency Virus. Journal of Virology 2001;75(7) 3371-3382.

[68] Atkinson H, Chalmers R. Delivering the Goods: Viral and Non-Viral Gene Therapy Systems and the Inherent Limits on Cargo DNA and Internal Sequences. Genetica 2010;138(5) 485-498.

[69] Chen Y, Du D, Wu J, Chan CP, Tan Y, Kung HF, He ML. Inhibition of Hepatitis B Virus Replication by Stably Expressed shRNA. Biochemical and Biophysical Research Communications 2003;311(2) 398-404.

[70] Kumar A, Panda SK, Durgapal H, Acharya SK, Rehman S, Kar UK. Inhibition of Hepatitis E Virus Replication Using Short Hairpin RNA (shRNA). Antiviral Research 2010;85(3) 541-550.

[71] Bushman FD. Retroviral Integration and Human Gene Therapy. Journal of Clinical Investigation 2007;117(8) 2083-2086.

[72] Brummelkamp TR, Bernards R, Agami R. Stable Suppression of Tumorigenicity by Virus-Mediated RNA Interference. Cancer Cell 2002;2(3) 243-247.

[73] Anesti AM, Peeters PJ, Royaux I, Coffin RS. Efficient Delivery of RNA Interference to Peripheral Neurons in Vivo Using Herpes Simplex Virus. Nucleic Acids Research 2008;36(14).

[74] Manjunath N, Wu H, Subramanya S, Shankar P. Lentiviral Delivery of Short Hairpin RNAs. Advanced Drug Delivery Reviews 2009;61(9) 732-745.

[75] Carlson ME, Hsu M, Conboy IM. Imbalance between Psmad3 and Notch Induces Cdk Inhibitors in Old Muscle Stem Cells. Nature 2008;454(7203) 528-532.

[76] Yoo JY, Kim JH, Kwon YG, Kim EC, Kim NK, Choi HJ, Yun CO. Vegf-Specific Short Hairpin RNA-Expressing Oncolytic Adenovirus Elicits Potent Inhibition of Angiogenesis and Tumor Growth. Molecular Therapy 2007;15(2) 295-302.

[77] Xia H, Mao Q, Eliason SL, Harper SQ, Martins IH, Orr HT, Paulson HL, Yang L, Kotin RM, Davidson BL. RNAi Suppresses Polyglutamine-Induced Neurodegeneration in a Model of Spinocerebellar Ataxia. Nature Medicine 2004;10(8) 816-820.

[78] Kuhlmann KF, Gouma DJ, Wesseling JG. Adenoviral Gene Therapy for Pancreatic Cancer: Where Do We Stand? Digestive Surgery 2008;25(4) 278-292.

[79] Descamps D, Benihoud K. Two Key Challenges for Effective Adenovirus-Mediated Liver Gene Therapy: Innate Immune Responses and Hepatocyte-Specific Transduction. Current Gene Therapy 2009;9(2) 115-127.

[80] Nayak S, Herzog RW. Progress and Prospects: Immune Responses to Viral Vectors. Gene Therapy 2010;17(3) 295-304.

[81] Raper SE, Chirmule N, Lee FS, Wivel NA, Bagg A, Gao GP, Wilson JM, Batshaw ML. Fatal Systemic Inflammatory Response Syndrome in a Ornithine Transcarbamylase Deficient Patient Following Adenoviral Gene Transfer. Molecular Genetics and Metabolism 2003;80(1-2) 148-158.

[82] Howe SJ, Mansour MR, Schwarzwaelder K, Bartholomae C, Hubank M, Kempski H, Brugman MH, Pike-Overzet K, Chatters SJ, de Ridder D, Gilmour KC, Adams S, Thornhill SI, Parsley KL, Staal FJ, Gale RE, Linch DC, Bayford J, Brown L, Quaye M, Kinnon C, Ancliff P, Webb DK, Schmidt M, von Kalle C, Gaspar HB, Thrasher AJ. Insertional Mutagenesis Combined with Acquired Somatic Mutations Causes Leuke-

mogenesis Following Gene Therapy of Scid-X1 Patients. Journal of Clinical Investigation 2008;118(9) 3143-3150.

[83] Hacein-Bey-Abina S, von Kalle C, Schmidt M, Le Deist F, Wulffraat N, McIntyre E, Radford I, Villeval JL, Fraser CC, Cavazzana-Calvo M, Fischer A. A Serious Adverse Event after Successful Gene Therapy for X-Linked Severe Combined Immunodeficiency. New England Journal of Medicine 2003;348(3) 255-256.

[84] Qasim W, Gaspar HB, Thrasher AJ. Progress and Prospects: Gene Therapy for Inherited Immunodeficiencies. Gene Therapy 2009;16(11) 1285-1291.

[85] Sheridan C. Gene Therapy Finds Its Niche. Nature Biotechnology 2011;29(2) 121-128.

[86] Mintzer MA, Simanek EE. Nonviral Vectors for Gene Delivery. Chemical Reviews 2009;109(2) 259-302.

[87] Torchilin VP, Rammohan R, Weissig V, Levchenko TS. Tat Peptide on the Surface of Liposomes Affords Their Efficient Intracellular Delivery Even at Low Temperature and in the Presence of Metabolic Inhibitors. Proceedings of the National Academy of Sciences of the United States of America 2001;98(15) 8786-8791.

[88] Torchilin VP, Levchenko TS, Rammohan R, Volodina N, Papahadjopoulos-Sternberg B, D'Souza GG. Cell Transfection in Vitro and in Vivo with Nontoxic Tat Peptide-Liposome-DNA Complexes. Proceedings of the National Academy of Sciences of the United States of America 2003;100(4) 1972-1977.

[89] Snyder EL, Dowdy SF. Cell Penetrating Peptides in Drug Delivery. Pharmaceutical Research 2004;21(3) 389-393.

[90] Gait MJ. Peptide-Mediated Cellular Delivery of Antisense Oligonucleotides and Their Analogues. Cellular and Molecular Life Sciences 2003;60(5) 844-853.

[91] Eguchi A, Akuta T, Okuyama H, Senda T, Yokoi H, Inokuchi H, Fujita S, Hayakawa T, Takeda K, Hasegawa M, Nakanishi M. Protein Transduction Domain of HIV-1 Tat Protein Promotes Efficient Delivery of DNA into Mammalian Cells. Journal of Biological Chemistry 2001;276(28) 26204-26210.

[92] Foerg C, Merkle HP. On the Biomedical Promise of Cell Penetrating Peptides: Limits Versus Prospects. Journal of Pharmaceutical Sciences 2008;97(1) 144-162.

[93] Mäe M, Andaloussi SE, Lehto T, Langel Ü. Chemically Modified Cell-Penetrating Peptides for the Delivery of Nucleic Acids. Expert Opinion on Drug Delivery 2009;6(11) 1195-1205.

[94] Crombez L, Aldrian-Herrada G, Konate K, Nguyen QN, McMaster GK, Brasseur R, Heitz F, Divita G. A New Potent Secondary Amphipathic Cell-Penetrating Peptide for siRNA Delivery into Mammalian Cells. Molecular Therapy 2009;17(1) 95-103.

[95] Lundberg P, El-Andaloussi S, Sutlu T, Johansson H, Langel U. Delivery of Short Interfering RNA Using Endosomolytic Cell-Penetrating Peptides. FASEB Journal
2007;21(11) 2664-2671.

[96] Simeoni F, Morris MC, Heitz F, Divita G. Insight into the Mechanism of the Peptide-
Based Gene Delivery System Mpg: Implications for Delivery of siRNA into Mammalian Cells. Nucleic Acids Research 2003;31(11) 2717-2724.

[97] Zeineddine D, Papadimou E, Chebli K, Gineste M, Liu J, Grey C, Thurig S, Behfar A,
Wallace VA, Skerjanc IS, Puceat M. Oct-3/4 Dose Dependently Regulates Specifica-
tion of Embryonic Stem Cells toward a Cardiac Lineage and Early Heart Development. Developmental Cell 2006;11(4) 535-546.

[98] Kim WJ, Christensen LV, Jo S, Yockman JW, Jeong JH, Kim YH, Kim SW. Cholesteryl
Oligoarginine Delivering Vascular Endothelial Growth Factor siRNA Effectively Inhibits Tumor Growth in Colon Adenocarcinoma. Molecular Therapy 2006;14(3)
343-350.

[99] Davidson TJ, Harel S, Arboleda VA, Prunell GF, Shelanski ML, Greene LA, Troy CM.
Highly Efficient Small Interfering RNA Delivery to Primary Mammalian Neurons Induces microRNA-Like Effects before mRNA Degradation. Journal of Neuroscience
2004;24(45) 10040-10046.

[100] Turner JJ, Jones S, Fabani MM, Ivanova G, Arzumanov AA, Gait MJ. RNA Targeting
with Peptide Conjugates of Oligonucleotides, siRNA and Pna. Blood Cells, Molecules, and Diseases 2007;38(1) 1-7.

[101] Chiu YL, Ali A, Chu CY, Cao H, Rana TM. Visualizing a Correlation between siRNA
Localization, Cellular Uptake, and RNAi in Living Cells. Chemistry and Biology
2004;11(8) 1165-1175.

[102] Frankel AD, Pabo CO. Cellular Uptake of the Tat Protein from Human Immunodeficiency Virus. Cell 1988;55(6) 1189-1193.

[103] Vives E, Brodin P, Lebleu B. A Truncated HIV-1 Tat Protein Basic Domain Rapidly
Translocates through the Plasma Membrane and Accumulates in the Cell Nucleus.
Journal of Biological Chemistry 1997;272(25) 16010-16017.

[104] Jones AT. Macropinocytosis: Searching for an Endocytic Identity and Role in the Uptake of Cell Penetrating Peptides. Journal of Cellular and Molecular Medicine
2007;11(4) 670-684.

[105] Patel LN, Zaro JL, Shen WC. Cell Penetrating Peptides: Intracellular Pathways and
Pharmaceutical Perspectives. Pharmaceutical Research 2007;24(11) 1977-1992.

[106] Hassani Z, Lemkine GF, Erbacher P, Palmier K, Alfama G, Giovannangeli C, Behr JP,
Demeneix BA. Lipid-Mediated siRNA Delivery Down-Regulates Exogenous Gene
Expression in the Mouse Brain at Picomolar Levels. The Journal of Gene Medicine
2005;7(2) 198-207.

[107]  Grayson AC, Doody AM, Putnam D. Biophysical and Structural Characterization of Polyethylenimine-Mediated siRNA Delivery in Vitro. Pharmaceutical Research 2006;23(8) 1868-1876.

[108]  Spagnou S, Miller AD, Keller M. Lipidic Carriers of siRNA: Differences in the Formulation, Cellular Uptake, and Delivery with Plasmid DNA. Biochemistry 2004;43(42) 13348-13356.

[109]  Bolcato-Bellemin AL, Bonnet ME, Creusatt G, Erbacher P, Behr JP. Sticky Overhangs Enhance siRNA-Mediated Gene Silencing. Proceedings of the National Academy of Sciences of the United States of America 2007;104 16050-16055.

[110]  Moghimi SM, Symonds P, Murray JC, Hunter AC, Debska G, Szewczyk A. A Two-Stage Poly(Ethylenimine)-Mediated Cytotoxicity: Implications for Gene Transfer/Therapy. Molecular Therapy 2005;11(6) 990-995.

[111]  Werth S, Urban-Klein B, Dai L, Hobel S, Grzelinski M, Bakowsky U, Czubayko F, Aigner A. A Low Molecular Weight Fraction of Polyethylenimine (PEI) Displays Increased Transfection Efficiency of DNA and siRNA in Fresh or Lyophilized Complexes. Journal of Controlled Release 2006;112(2) 257-270. DOI: 10.1016/j.jconrel.2006.02.009.

[112]  Boussif O, Lezoualc'h F, Zanta MA, Mergny MD, Scherman D, Demeneix B, Behr JP. A Versatile Vector for Gene and Oligonucleotide Transfer into Cells in Culture and in Vivo: Polyethylenimine. Proceedings of the National Academy of Sciences of the United States of America 1995;92(16) 7297-7301.

[113]  Philipp A, Zhao X, Tarcha P, Wagner E, Zintchenko A. Hydrophobically Modified Oligoethylenimines as Highly Efficient Transfection Agents for siRNA Delivery. Bioconjugate Chemistry 2009;20(11) 2055-2061.

[114]  Bajaj A, Kondaiah P, Bhattacharya S. Synthesis and Gene Transfection Efficacies of PEI-Cholesterol-Based Lipopolymers. Bioconjugate Chemistry 2008;19(8) 1640-1651.

[115]  Breunig M, Hozsa C, Lungwitz U, Watanabe K, Umeda I, Kato H, Goepferich A. Mechanistic Investigation of Poly(Ethyleneimine)-Based siRNA Delivery: Disulfide Bonds Boost Intracellular Release of the Cargo. Journal of Controlled Release 2008;130(1) 57-63.

[116]  Mao S, Sun W, Kissel T. Chitosan-Based Formulations for Delivery of DNA and siRNA. Advanced Drug Delivery Reviews 2010;62(1) 12-27.

[117]  Liu X, Howard KA, Dong M, Andersen MO, Rahbek UL, Johnsen MG, Hansen OC, Besenbacher F, Kjems J. The Influence of Polymeric Properties on Chitosan/siRNA Nanoparticle Formulation and Gene Silencing. Biomaterials 2007;28(6) 1280-1288.

[118]  Katas H, Alpar HO. Development and Characterisation of Chitosan Nanoparticles for siRNA Delivery. Journal of Controlled Release 2006;115(2) 216-225.

[119]  Menuel S, Fontanay S, Clarot I, Duval RE, Diez L, Marsura A. Synthesis and Complexation Ability of a Novel Bis-(Guanidinium)-Tetrakis-(Beta-Cyclodextrin) Dendri-
meric Tetrapod as a Potential Gene Delivery (DNA and siRNA) System. Study of
Cellular siRNA Transfection. Bioconjugate Chemistry 2008;19(12) 2357-2362.

[120]  Hu-Lieskovan S, Heidel JD, Bartlett DW, Davis ME, Triche TJ. Sequence-Specific
Knockdown of Ews-Fli1 by Targeted, Nonviral Delivery of Small Interfering RNA Inhibits Tumor Growth in a Murine Model of Metastatic Ewing's Sarcoma. Cancer Research 2005;65(19) 8984-8992.

[121]  Davis ME. The First Targeted Delivery of siRNA in Humans Via a Self-Assembling,
Cyclodextrin Polymer-Based Nanoparticle: From Concept to Clinic. Molecular Pharmaceutics 2009;6(3) 659-668.

[122]  Davis ME, Zuckerman JE, Choi CH, Seligson D, Tolcher A, Alabi CA, Yen Y, Heidel
JD, Ribas A. Evidence of RNAi in Humans from Systemically Administered siRNA
Via Targeted Nanoparticles. Nature 2010;464(7291) 1067-1070.

[123]  O'Mahony AM, Ogier J, Desgranges S, Cryan JF, Darcy R, O'Driscoll CM. A Click
Chemistry Route to 2-Functionalised Pegylated and Cationic Beta-Cyclodextrins: Co-
Formulation Opportunities for siRNA Delivery. Organic and Biomolecular Chemis-
try 2012;10(25) 4954-4960.

[124]  Zhu L, Mahato RI. Lipid and Polymeric Carrier-Mediated Nucleic Acid Delivery. Expert Opinion on Drug Delivery 2010;7(10) 1209-1226.

[125]  Dufès C, Uchegbu IF, Schätzlein AG. Dendrimers in Gene Delivery. Advanced Drug
Delivery Reviews 2005;57(15) 2177-2202.

[126]  Zinselmeyer BH, Mackay SP, Schatzlein AG, Uchegbu IF. The Lower-Generation Polypropylenimine Dendrimers Are Effective Gene-Transfer Agents. Pharmaceutical
Research 2002;19(7) 960-967.

[127]  Fischer D, Li Y, Ahlemeyer B, Krieglstein J, Kissel T. In Vitro Cytotoxicity Testing of
Polycations: Influence of Polymer Structure on Cell Viability and Hemolysis. Biomaterials 2003;24(7) 1121-1131.

[128]  Sonawane ND, Szoka FC, Verkman AS. Chloride Accumulation and Swelling in Endosomes Enhances DNA Transfer by Polyamine-DNA Polyplexes. Journal of Biological Chemistry 2003;278(45) 44826-44831.

[129]  Taratula O, Savla R, He HX, Minko T. Poly(Propyleneimine) Dendrimers as Potential
siRNA Delivery Nanocarrier: From Structure to Function. International Journal of
Nanotechnology 2011;8(1-2) 36-52.

[130]  Perez AP, Romero EL, Morilla MJ. Ethylendiamine Core PAMAM Dendrimers/
siRNA Complexes as in Vitro Silencing Agents. International Journal of Pharmaceutics 2009;380(1-2) 189-200.

[131]  Felgner PL, Gadek TR, Holm M, Roman R, Chan HW, Wenz M, Northrop JP, Ring-old GM, Danielsen M. Lipofection: A Highly Efficient, Lipid-Mediated DNA-Trans-fection Procedure. Proceedings of the National Academy of Sciences of the United States of America 1987;84(21) 7413-7417.

[132]  Martin B, Sainlos M, Aissaoui A, Oudrhiri N, Hauchecorne M, Vigneron JP, Lehn JM, Lehn P. The Design of Cationic Lipids for Gene Delivery. Current Pharmaceutical Design 2005;11(3) 375-394.

[133]  Bhattacharya S, Bajaj A. Advances in Gene Delivery through Molecular Design of Cationic Lipids. Chemical Communications 2009;(31) 4632-4656.

[134]  Shirazi RS, Ewert KK, Leal C, Majzoub RN, Bouxsein NF, Safinya CR. Synthesis and Characterization of Degradable Multivalent Cationic Lipids with Disulfide-Bond Spacers for Gene Delivery. Biochimica et Biophysica Acta-Biomembranes 2011;1808(9) 2156-2166.

[135]  Guenin E, Herve AC, Floch V, Loisel S, Yaouanc JJ, Clement JC, Ferec C, des Abbayes H. Cationic Phosphonolipids Containing Quaternary Phosphonium and Arsonium Groups for DNA Transfection with Good Efficiency and Low Cellular Toxicity. An-gewandte Chemie International Edition 2000;39(3) 629-631.

[136]  Floch V, Loisel S, Guenin E, Herve AC, Clement JC, Yaouanc JJ, des Abbayes H, Fer-ec C. Cation Substitution in Cationic Phosphonolipids: A New Concept to Improve Transfection Activity and Decrease Cellular Toxicity. Journal of Medicinal Chemistry 2000;43(24) 4617-4628.

[137]  Hasegawa S, Hirashima N, Nakanishi M. Comparative Study of Transfection Effi-ciency of Cationic Cholesterols Mediated by Liposomes-Based Gene Delivery. Bioor-ganic and Medicinal Chemistry Letters 2002;12(9) 1299-1302.

[138]  Felgner JH, Kumar R, Sridhar CN, Wheeler CJ, Tsai YJ, Border R, Ramsey P, Martin M, Felgner PL. Enhanced Gene Delivery and Mechanism Studies with a Novel Series of Cationic Lipid Formulations. Journal of Biological Chemistry 1994;269(4) 2550-2561.

[139]  Bennett MJ, Aberle AM, Balasubramaniam RP, Malone JG, Malone RW, Nantz MH. Cationic Lipid-Mediated Gene Delivery to Murine Lung: Correlation of Lipid Hydra-tion with in Vivo Transfection Activity. Journal of Medicinal Chemistry 1997;40(25) 4069-4078.

[140]  Sen J, Chaudhuri A. Design, Syntheses, and Transfection Biology of Novel Non-Cho-lesterol-Based Guanidinylated Cationic Lipids. Journal of Medicinal Chemistry 2005;48(3) 812-820.

[141]  Gao H, Hui KM. Synthesis of a Novel Series of Cationic Lipids That Can Act as Effi-cient Gene Delivery Vehicles through Systematic Heterocyclic Substitution of Choles-terol Derivatives. Gene Therapy 2001;8(11) 855-863.

[142] Schmid N, Behr JP. Location of Spermine and Other Polyamines on DNA as Revealed by Photoaffinity Cleavage with Polyaminobenzenediazonium Salts. Biochemistry 1991;30(17) 4357-4361.

[143] Bernstein H-G, Müller M. The Cellular Localization of the L-Ornithine Decarboxylase/Polyamine System in Normal and Diseased Central Nervous Systems. Progress in Neurobiology 1999;57(5) 485-505.

[144] Janne J, Poso H, Raina A. Polyamines in Rapid Growth and Cancer. Biochimica et Biophysica Acta 1978;473(3-4) 241-293.

[145] Fozard JR, Part ML, Prakash NJ, Grove J, Schechter PJ, Sjoerdsma A, Koch-Weser J. L-Ornithine Decarboxylase: An Essential Role in Early Mammalian Embryogenesis. Science 1980;208(4443) 505-508.

[146] Pegg AE, Seely JE, Poso H, della Ragione F, Zagon IA. Polyamine Biosynthesis and Interconversion in Rodent Tissues. Federation Proceedings 1982;41(14) 3065-3072.

[147] Pegg AE, McCann PP. Polyamine Metabolism and Function. American Journal of Physiology 1982;243(5) C212-221.

[148] Janne J, Alhonen L, Leinonen P. Polyamines - from Molecular-Biology to Clinical-Applications. Annals of Medicine 1991;23(3) 241-259.

[149] Hougaard DM. Polyamine Cytochemistry: Localization and Possible Functions of Polyamines. International Review of Cytology 1992;138 51-88.

[150] Behr JP, Demeneix B, Loeffler JP, Perez-Mutul J. Efficient Gene Transfer into Mammalian Primary Endocrine Cells with Lipopolyamine-Coated DNA. Proceedings of the National Academy of Sciences of the United States of America 1989;86(18) 6982-6986.

[151] Moradpour D, Schauer JI, Zurawski VR, Wands JR, Boutin RH. Efficient Gene Transfer into Mammalian Cells with Cholesteryl-Spermidine. Biochemical and Biophysical Research Communications 1996;221(1) 82-88.

[152] Geall AJ, Eaton MAW, Baker T, Catterall C, Blagbrough IS. The Regiochemical Distribution of Positive Charges Along Cholesterol Polyamine Carbamates Plays Significant Roles in Modulating DNA Binding Affinity and Lipofection. FEBS Letters 1999;459(3) 337-342.

[153] Fujiwara T, Hasegawa S, Hirashima N, Nakanishi M, Ohwada T. Gene Transfection Activities of Amphiphilic Steroid-Polyamine Conjugates. Biochimica et Biophysica Acta-Biomembranes 2000;1468(1-2) 396-402.

[154] Koynova R, Tenchov B, Wang L, MacDonald RC. Hydrophobic Moiety of Cationic Lipids Strongly Modulates Their Transfection Activity. Molecular Pharmaceutics 2009;6(3) 951-958.

[155] Incani V, Lavasanifar A, Uludag H. Lipid and Hydrophobic Modification of Cationic Carriers on Route to Superior Gene Vectors. Soft Matter 2010;6(10) 2124-2138.

[156] Koynova R, Tenchov B. Cationic Phospholipids: Structure-Transfection Activity Relationships. Soft Matter 2009;5(17) 3187-3200.

[157] Floch V, Legros N, Loisel S, Guillaume C, Guilbot J, Benvegnu T, Ferrieres V, Plusquellec D, Ferec C. New Biocompatible Cationic Amphiphiles Derivative from Glycine Betaine: A Novel Family of Efficient Nonviral Gene Transfer Agents. Biochemical and Biophysical Research Communications 1998;251(1) 360-365.

[158] Wang J, Guo X, Xu Y, Barron L, Szoka FC, Jr. Synthesis and Characterization of Long Chain Alkyl Acyl Carnitine Esters. Potentially Biodegradable Cationic Lipids for Use in Gene Delivery. Journal of Medicinal Chemistry 1998;41(13) 2207-2215.

[159] Laxmi AA, Vijayalakshmi P, Kaimal TN, Chaudhuri A, Ramadas Y, Rao NM. Novel Non-Glycerol-Based Cytofectins with Lactic Acid-Derived Head Groups. Biochemical and Biophysical Research Communications 2001;289(5) 1057-1062.

[160] Heyes JA, Niculescu-Duvaz D, Cooper RG, Springer CJ. Synthesis of Novel Cationic Lipids: Effect of Structural Modification on the Efficiency of Gene Transfer. Journal of Medicinal Chemistry 2002;45(1) 99-114.

[161] Lindner LH, Brock R, Arndt-Jovin D, Eibl H. Structural Variation of Cationic Lipids: Minimum Requirement for Improved Oligonucleotide Delivery into Cells. Journal of Controlled Release 2006;110(2) 444-456.

[162] Xu YH, Szoka FC. Mechanism of DNA Release from Cationic Liposome/DNA Complexes Used in Cell Transfection. Biochemistry 1996;35(18) 5616-5623.

[163] Ghonaim HM, Ahmed OAA, Pourzand C, Blagbrough IS. Varying the Chain Length in $N^4,N^9$-Diacyl Spermines: Non-Viral Lipopolyamine Vectors for Efficient Plasmid DNA Formulation. Molecular Pharmaceutics 2008;5(6) 1111-1121.

[164] McGregor C, Perrin C, Monck M, Camilleri P, Kirby AJ. Rational Approaches to the Design of Cationic Gemini Surfactants for Gene Delivery. Journal of the American Chemical Society 2001;123(26) 6215-6220.

[165] Heyes J, Palmer L, Bremner K, MacLachlan I. Cationic Lipid Saturation Influences Intracellular Delivery of Encapsulated Nucleic Acids. Journal of Controlled Release 2005;107(2) 276-287.

[166] Hattori Y, Hagiwara A, Ding W, Maitani Y. Nacl Improves siRNA Delivery Mediated by Nanoparticles of Hydroxyethylated Cationic Cholesterol with Amido-Linker. Bioorganic and Medicinal Chemistry Letters 2008;18(19) 5228-5232.

[167] Rao NM, Gopal V. Cationic Lipids for Gene Delivery in Vitro and in Vivo. Expert Opinion on Therapeutic Patents 2006;16(6) 825-844.

[168] Ilies MA, Seitz WA, Johnson BH, Ezell EL, Miller AL, Thompson EB, Balaban AT. Lipophilic Pyrylium Salts in the Synthesis of Efficient Pyridinium-Based Cationic

Lipids, Gemini Surfactants, and Lipophilic Oligomers for Gene Delivery. Journal of Medicinal Chemistry 2006;49(13) 3872-3887.

[169] Zhu L, Lu Y, Miller DD, Mahato RI. Structural and Formulation Factors Influencing Pyridinium Lipid-Based Gene Transfer. Bioconjugate Chemistry 2008;19(12) 2499-2512.

[170] Medvedeva DA, Maslov MA, Serikov RN, Morozova NG, Serebrenikova GA, Sheglov DV, Latyshev AV, Vlassov VV, Zenkova MA. Novel Cholesterol-Based Cationic Lipids for Gene Delivery. Journal of Medicinal Chemistry 2009;52(21) 6558-6568.

[171] Guo X, Szoka FC. Chemical Approaches to Triggerable Lipid Vesicles for Drug and Gene Delivery. Accounts of Chemical Research 2003;36(5) 335-341.

[172] Chen HG, Zhang HZ, McCallum CM, Szoka FC, Guo X. Unsaturated Cationic Ortho Esters for Endosome Permeation in Gene Delivery. Journal of Medicinal Chemistry 2007;50(18) 4269-4278.

[173] Bajaj A, Kondaiah P, Bhattacharya S. Effect of the Nature of the Spacer on Gene Transfer Efficacies of Novel Thiocholesterol Derived Gemini Lipids in Different Cell Lines: A Structure-Activity Investigation. Journal of Medicinal Chemistry 2008;51(8) 2533-2540.

[174] Metwally AA, Pourzand C, Blagbrough IS. Efficient Gene Silencing by Self-assembled Complexes of siRNA and Symmetrical Fatty Acid Amides of Spermine, Pharmaceutics 2011;3 125-140. DOI: 10.3390/pharmaceutics3020125.

[175] Metwally AA, Blagbrough IS. Self-assembled Lipoplexes of Short Interfering RNA (siRNA) Using Spermine-based Fatty Acid Amide Guanidines: Effect on Gene Silencing Efficiency, Pharmaceutics 2011;3 406-424. DOI: 10.3390/pharmaceutics3030406.

[176] Blagbrough IS, Metwally AA, Ghonaim HM, Asymmetrical N4,N9-Diacyl Spermines: SAR studies of Nonviral Lipopolyamine Vectors for Efficient siRNA Delivery with Silencing of EGFP Reporter Gene, Molecular Pharmaceutics 2012;9 1853-1861.

[177] Metwally AA, Reelfs O, Pourzand C, Blagbrough IS, Efficient Silencing of EGFP Reporter Gene with siRNA Delivered by Asymmetrical N4,N9-Diacyl Spermines, Molecular Pharmaceutics 2012;9 1862-1876.

[178] Metwally AA, Blagbrough IS, Mantell JM, Quantitative Silencing of EGFP Reporter Gene by Self-assembled siRNA Lipoplexes of LinOS and Cholesterol, Molecular Pharmaceutics, 2012;9 3384-3395. DOI: 10.1021/mp300435x.

[179] Nguyen DN, Mahon KP, Chikh G, Kim P, Chung H, Vicari AP, Love KT, Goldberg M, Chen S, Krieg AM, Chen JZ, Langer R, Anderson DG. Lipid-derived Nanoparticles for Immunostimulatory RNA Adjuvant Delivery. Proceedings of the National Academy of Sciences of the United States of America 2012;109(14) E797-E803. DOI: 10.1073/pnas.1121423109.

[180] Lee H, Lytton-Jean AKR, Chen Y, Love KT, Park AI, Karagiannis ED, Sehgal A, Querbes W, Zurenko CS, Jayaraman M, Peng CG, Charisse K, Borodovsky A, Manoharan M, Donahoe JS, Truelove J, Nahrendorf M, Langer R, Anderson DG. Molecularly Self-assembled Nucleic Acid Nanoparticles for Targeted in Vivo siRNA Delivery. Nature Nanotechnology 2012;7(6) 389-393. DOI: 10.1038/NNANO.2012.73.

[181] Geall AJ, Verma A, Otten GR, Shaw CA, Hekele A, Banerjee K, Cu Y, Beard CW, Brito LA, Krucker T, O'Hagan DT, Singh M, Mason PW, Valiante NM, Dormitzer PR, Barnett SW, Rappuoli R, Ulmer JB, Mandl CW. Nonviral Delivery of Self-amplifying RNA Vaccines. Proceedings of the National Academy of Sciences of the United States of America 2012;109(36) 14604-14609. DOI: 10.1073/pnas.1209367109.

[182] Duan S, Yuan W, Wu F, Jin T. Polyspermine Imidazole-4,5-imine, a Chemically Dynamic and Biologically Responsive Carrier System for Intracellular Delivery of siRNA. Angewandte Chemie International Edition 2012;51(32), 7938-7941. DOI: 10.1002/anie.201201793.

# Chapter 6

# Cellular Uptake Mechanism of Non-Viral Gene Delivery and Means for Improving Transfection Efficiency

Shengnan Xiang and Xiaoling Zhang

Additional information is available at the end of the chapter

## 1. Introduction

Non-viral delivery systems usually include mechanical, electrical, and chemical methods. Cationic liposomes and cationic polymers are two typical classes of non-viral vectors. Compared with viral vectors, non-viral ones are considered promising vehicles for gene therapy because of their low toxicity, biocompatibility, and controllability [1, 2], although their low efficacy limits their application as a mature gene delivery system. Improving the efficacy of non-viral vectors necessitates thorough understanding of their *in vivo* key steps. Non-viral vectors can complex with gene materials and help them access the target compartments within cells. Many barriers prevent gene materials from reaching their intended target and performing their functions [3], safe and effective delivery remains an important challenge for the clinical development of non-viral vectors [4].

The delivery of pDNA or siRNA *in vivo* for therapeutic aims has been widely studied in recent years. However, non-viral delivery systems, which exhibit relatively low levels of efficiency, are not clinically applicable. Improving their efficiency is the main task of pDNA- or siRNA-based gene therapy. There are many barriers that hinder pDNA and siRNA from reaching their intended target in the plasma and performing their functions: First, gene materials can be loaded into vectors. After *in vivo* administration, the vectors must be delivered to the blood vessels and should be stable in the blood; otherwise, they will be cleared by albumin because of their high surface charge and may also be uptaken by macrophages. The vectors must then pass through the epithelial tissue of the blood vessels and enter the target tissue. As it is very difficult for nanoparticles larger than 5 nm in diameter to pass through the epithelial tissue of blood vessels [5], it is crucial to study the cellular transport mechanism of epithelial cells through the caveolin-mediated endocytosis (CvME) pathway which is active in epithelial cells [6]. The distance between the extracellular matrix and target cells is great, and many vectors will be uptaken and cleared by macrophages after they do manage to pass through the epithelial tissue of blood vessels.

Next, the vectors must attach to the cell membrane, which entails other issues altogether. First, the non-viral vectors should be able to identify specific cell types to ensure safety. They then enter cells mainly via endocytosis. Different endocytosis pathways yield different intracellular fates for vectors, which could potentially explain why the same vector differs in its transfection efficiency in various cell modes. After their entry into the cells, vectors must escape from the endosome or avoid the endo-lysosomal (endosomal and lysosomal) pathway through certain endocytosis pathways. After escaping the endosome and then entering the cytoplasm, vectors must release pDNA or siRNA and finally perform their function in the cytoplasm [5]. In addition, pDNA has to be transported into the nucleus. The key steps in non-viral delivery are shown in Figure 1.

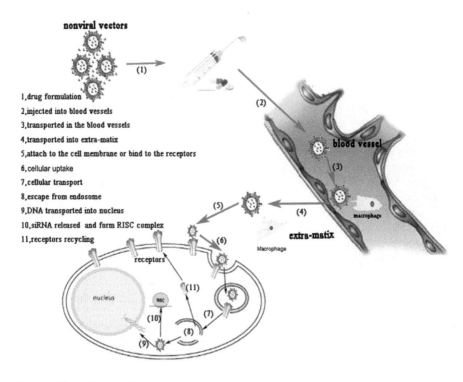

**Figure 1.** Biological key steps of non-viral vectors

As discussed above, the cellular process (including uptake, transport, endosomal escape, and nuclear localization) is one of the most important steps for non-viral gene delivery. In 2001, Hideyoshi Harashima et al. stated that novel strategies of medical treatments, such as gene therapy, highlight the importance of studying the intracellular fate of macromolecules, such as DNA and siRNA. In particular, in the case of gene therapy, intracellular events would be expected to be the major factors controlling the fate of the introduced gene and the efficiency of its expression. These authors attempted to establish an intracellular pharmaco-kinetic model of genes to study the intracellular events involved in gene therapy [7]. Under-standing the intracellular fate of a gene or vector is important for us to overcome the cellular barriers of DNA or siRNA delivery and rationally design efficient systems thereof.

Of all intracellular events, the cellular uptake mechanism of non-viral vectors is the most es-sential to their efficiency and intracellular fate. Different cellular uptake pathways have dif-ferent intracellular fates. As the gene materials will be degraded in the endo-lysosomes (endosomes and lysosomes). One good example is that some endocytic pathways involve endo-lysosomes, but others that can bypass the endo-lysosomes have higher levels of deliv-ery efficiency. Polyethylenimine (PEI) is one of the most promising non-viral vectors [8]. Some researchers have shown that cellular uptake of PEI polyplexes affects other cellular processes and, consequently, transfection efficiency [9, 10]. These differences may depend on such factors as the size, surface properties, and shape of the particles [11], as well as dif-ferent cell lines [9].

Research has shown that polyplexes and lipoplexes have different uptake mechanisms in A549 pneumocytes and HeLa cells. Lipoplex uptake proceeds only by clathrin-mediated en-docytosis (CME), whereas polyplexes are taken up by two mechanisms — one involving caveolae and another using clathrin-coated pits [10]. As the caveolae-mediated uptake mechanism has slower kinetics, the transfection process of polyplexes is slower than that of lipoplexes in A549 pneumocytes and HeLa cells. However, as the polyplexes uptaken via the caveolae escape the lysosomal compartment, polyplexes have a high level of transfection efficiency [10]. Taken together, these findings highlight the importance of studying the cellu-lar uptake of non-viral vectors, their intracellular fate, and their effects on transfection effi-ciency. Understanding cellular uptake mechanisms is crucial to engineering successful reagents or vectors for non-viral gene transfection [12].

## 2. Cellular uptake pathways of non-viral gene delivery

The uptake pathways are divided into two groups: endocytic pathways and non-endocytic pathways. Inside endocytic group, there are two types of pathways: phagocytosis and non-phagocytosis pathways [11].

### 2.1. Phagocytosis

Phagocytosis is a special type of endocytic pathway which primarily exists in professional phagocytes such as macrophages, monocytes neutrophils, and dendritic cells (DCs) [13]. In comparison, other nonphagocytic pathways such as clathrin-mediated endocytosis (CME), caveolae-mediated endocytosis (CvME), and macropinocytosis occur in almost all kinds of cell types [14]. Phagocytic pathway is mediated by cup-like membrane extensions that are usually larger than 1 μm to internalize large particles such as bacteria or dead cells. Under-standing of the mechanism of phagocytosis is very helpful to the non-viral gene therapy of macrophage-dominated immune diseases such as rheumatoid arthritis. In addition, a phag-ocytosis-like mechanism was proposed for the uptake of large lipoplexes and polyplexes that are larger than can be taken up by the classic CME pathway [15, 16].

Phagocytosis depending on opsonins can be called as opsonic phagocytosis. There is also another phagocytosis which is opsonins independent. This will be discussed later. First, for opsonic phagocytosis, the complexes will be recognized by opsonins in the bloodstream. Then, the opsonized complexes adhere to professional phagocytes and are ultimately ingest-ed by them [11]. Opsonization is the key step of the phagocytosis pathway. It involves com-plexes tagged by some major opsonins including immunoglobulins G and M (IgG and IgM), as well as complement components C3, C4, and C5 in the bloodstream [11, 17]. These opson-ized complexes become visible to macrophages and bind to their surface through the inter-action between receptors (such as fragment crystallizable receptors (FcR) and complement receptors (CR)) and the constant fragment of particle-adsorbed immunoglobulins.

Other receptors that mediate phagocytosis pathway have also been reported. Mannose re-ceptor (MR) has been used in gene vaccine by targeting human DCs and macrophages through the phagocytic pathway [18]. Scavenger receptor (SR)-mediated delivery of anti-sense miniexon phosphorothioate oligonucleotide to leishmania-infected macrophages is proved to be selective and efficient in eliminating the parasite [19]. SR-A, macrophage recep-tor, and CD36 are the three SR subtypes. CD36 can mediate non-opsonic phagocytosis of pathogenic microbes [20]. Unlike opsonic phagocytosis, non-opsonic phagocytosis is directly mediated by the receptors on the cell surface without the help of opsonins. This kind of mechanism can also be used for gene delivery.

Then the activated Rho-family GTPases trigger actin assembly and cell surface extension for-mation. This surface extension finally zippers up around the complexes and engulfs them [11]. The phagosomes carrying the complexes fuse with lysosomes to form mature phagoly-sosomes [11]. In phagolysosomes, the complexes undergo a process of acidification and en-zymatic reaction. As the intracellular fate of phagocytosis is the transportation of complexes into the lysosome, the gene materials will be degraded by the nucleases inside it [21]. Endo-somes and lysosomes (endo-lysosomes) are very important biological barrier for gene deliv-ery. The vectors should have capability to escape form them, if gene materials loaded vectors entry into the cell via phagocytosis. The mechanisms of endo-lysosome escape will be discussed later.

## 2.2. Non- phagocytosis pathways

Non- phagocytosis pathways mainly include clathrin-mediated endocytosis (CME), caveo-lae-mediated endocytosis (CvME), and macropinocytosis. CME is the best-characterized type of endocytosis, which is receptor-dependent, clathrin-mediated, and GTPase dynamin-required [22, 23]. The uptake of low-density lipoprotein and transferrin is typically via this endocytic pathway, and they are often used as the CME probes in many studies [24, 25]. Transferrin has also been used as a ligand of non-viral vectors to improve the endocytosis of complexes [26, 27]. In this pathway, a series of downstream events are activated after the recognition of ligands by receptors on the cell surface. Clathrins assemble in the polyhedral lattice right on the cytosolic surface of the cell membrane, which helps to deform the membrane into a coated pit with a size about 100–150 nm [27]. This process is mediated by GTPase dynamin. As the clathrin lattice formation continues, the pit becomes deeply invaginated until the vesicle fission occurs. In the next step of the CME pathway, the endocytosed vesicles internalized from the plasma membrane are integrated into late endosomes and finally transported to lysosomes.

CvME begins in a special flask-shaped structure on the cell membrane called caveola, which is a kind of cholesterol- and sphingolipidrich smooth invagination [28]. CvME usually happens in the vessel wall lining monolayer of endothelial cells [7]. Caveolae have a diameter range of 50–100 nm [11] and are typically between 50 and 80 nmwith a neck of 10–50 nm [6]. CvME is also a type of cholesterol, dynamin-dependent, and receptor-mediated pathway [29]. The fission of the caveolae from the membrane is mediated by the GTPase dynamin, which locates in the neck of caveolae and then generates the cytosolic caveolar vesicle [11]. Some receptors located in caveolae, such as insulin receptors [30] and epidermal growth factor receptor (a type of receptor in ovarian cancer) [31], can mediate CvME [32]. The vesicle budding from the caveolae, a type of caveolin-1-containing endosome is called caveosome [29]. The intracellular fate of the caveosome differs from that of CME. Compared with CME, CvME is generally considered as a alternative pathway which can deliver the vectors into Golgi and/or endoplasmic reticulum, thus avoiding the normal lysosomal degradation

Macropinocytosis is a type of distinct pathway that nonspecifically takes up a large amount of fluid-phase contents through the mode called fluid-phase endocytosis (FPE) [33]. Macropinocytosis is a signal dependent process that normally occurs when macrophages or cancer cells are in response to colony-stimulating factor-1 (CSF-1), epidermal growth factor (EGF) and platelet-derived growth factor or tumor-promoting factor, such as phorbol myristate acetate respectively [34-36]. However, this process occurs constitutively in antigen-presenting cells [37]. Macropinocytosis occurs via the formation of actin-driven membrane protrusions, which is similar to phagocytosis. However, in this case, the protrusions do not zipper up the ligand-coated particle; instead, they collapse onto and fuse with the plasma membrane [11]. The macropinosomes have no apparent coat structures and are heterogenous in size, but are generally considered larger than 0.2 μm in diameter [38, 39]. During this process, the small GTPase, Ras-related in brain (Rab) proteins are essential for the vesicle fission from the cell membrane [40]. The relationship between the macropinocytosis and lysosome is still unknown. This will be discussed later.

## 2.3. Non-endocytic pathways

There are three technologies that are designed to mediate the non-endocytic pathways and successful transfect the gene. One is microinjection, by which each cell is injected with the gene materials using glass capillary pipettes. The second one is permeabilization by using pore-forming reagents such as streptolysin O or anionic peptides such as HA2 subunit of the influenza virus hemagglutinin. The third one is electroporation, which uses an electric field to open pores in the cell. All of them are highly invasive and not ideal for in vivo gene delivery.

However, There are evidences which can prove the existing of other non-endocytic pathways. One pathway is related to the formation of holes in the cell membrane, called "penetration". A class of cationic peptides with the protein transduction domains (PTDs), such as TAT, has the ability to be taken up without endocytic events [41]. These peptides can directly penetrate cell membranes in a receptor-, and energy-independent way. In 2004, Hong et al. studied the hole formation on the cell membrane induced by poly(amidoamine) (PAMAM). The results indicated that the hole formation can be induced by positively charged PAMAM, and labeled PAMAM can diffuse into the cells through small holes in the membrane. This mechanism is considered a nonspecific pathway, which is not receptor-mediated and lacks selective cellular uptake [42]. In 2010, Lee et al. used a PTD called Hph-1 to conjugate vector PEI to deliver siRNA. The result showed that the complexes entered the cells through the non-endocytic pathway, which has a quicker dynamic behavior compared with the endocytosis pathways and is energy-independent because it has high transfection efficiency even in low temperature [43]. Another non-endocytic pathway is called "fusion", which is special for lipoplexes, as it can cause a direct release of DNA to the cytoplasm before entering the endocytic pathways. However, more and more evidences suggest that fusion with the cell membrane contributes minimally to the overall uptake of lipoplexes, while the CME plays an important role in the uptake of lipoplexes [44]. there have been few studies on non-endocytic pathways, and more efforts are needed to have a comprehensive understanding of these pathways for the improvement of non-viral gene delivery.

| Pathways | GTPases | Relationship with lysosome | Receptors |
|---|---|---|---|
| Phagocytosis | Rho | Dependent | Dependent |
| CME | Dynamin | Dependent | Dependent |
| CvME | Dynamin | Independent | Dependent |
| Macropinocytosis | Rab | In dispute | Non-specific |
| Non-endocytic | Independent | Independent | Non-specific |

**Table 1.** Cellular uptake mechanisms.

## 3. Factors that influence the uptake pathways of non-viral gene delivery

There are many factors that are involved in the selection of uptake pathways of non-viral gene complexes. These factors include particle size, particle surface charge, particle shape, cell type, and even culture condition. Because the complexes of non-viral gene vector/DNA or siRNA are usually a group of heterogeneous particles with diverse sizes, surface charges, and shapes, several uptake pathways may be involved in the internalization of one kind of complexes into a single cell type. For example, transfection by branched PEI25kDa/DNA polyplexes was mediated by both CME and CvME pathways in HUH-7 and Hela cells [9]. Later, Hansjörg Hufnagel reported that the macropinocytosis is also very important for the uptake of branched PEI25kDa/DNA polyplexes into Hela and CHO-1 cells due to the existence of large particles of polyplexes (>500 nm) [12]. Therefore, the heterogeneity of complexes has to be taken into consideration when the results are analyzed. Particle size is a very important factor for the pathway selection of complexes. As mentioned above, the labeled cationic PAMAM can induce hole formation in the cell membrane. The holes induced by PAMAM are 15–40 nm in diameter [42]. The particle including the gene complex, which is smaller than these holes, can diffuse through the holes and be taken up by nonspecific non-endocytic rather than specific receptor mediated endocytic pathways. PEI/DNA complexes with sizes smaller than 500 nm are mainly taken up by CME and CvME according to a previous study [10]. While PEI/DNA complexes with sizes >500 nm are mainly internalized by macropinocytosis pathway [10].

The charge density of a complex is also an important factor for its uptake. The cell membrane consists of a bilayer of lipid and anionic membrane proteins. These anionic proteins are very helpful to the uptake of cationic complexes. However, once the net positive charge falls to neutral, the uptake efficiency will be inhibited a lot. This is because the neutral charge density will weaken the interaction between complexes and membrane proteins, and it will also increase the aggregation of complexes, which will make them large and hard to be internalized. This change can be caused by the anionic proteins in the in vivo circulation of blood, and the serum used in the in vitro transfection medium. The modification of polyethylene glycol (PEG) can solve this problem with its high hydrophilicity, electrical neutrality and steric-repulsive propensity [45].

As to the relationship between the shape of particles and the pathway selection, few studies have been made about this issue. A group once reported that the uptake of protein-coated spherical gold nanoparticles is more efficient than rod-shaped ones in Hela cells, SNB19 cells, and STO cells [46, 47]. However, as to the relationship of nonviral gene complexes and their uptake efficiency, it is not easy to draw such a conclusion, because the non-viral gene complexes are usually a group of nanoparticles with heterogeneous shapes, and their shapes are dependent on the experimental conditions. Taking chitosan as an example, the fraction of complexes that have nonaggregated, globular structures increases with increasing chain length of the chitosan oligomer, increasing charge ratio and reduction of pH (from 6.5 to 3.5) [48]. Because of this, this complicated issue leaves much room for researchers to discuss.

Cell type is another important factor that influences the pathway selection of non-viral gene complexes. Different types of cells can take up a kind of complex in different pathways. Most of the studies focused on COS-7 cells, which were used as a well-established model cell for gene delivery researches [28]. Some researchers also used other cell lines such as A549, Hela, and HUH-7 cells. Caveolae, which are a very important structure for CvME pathway, are present in many cell types, but they are particularly abundant in the vessel wall lining monolayer of endothelial cells. As a result, endothelial cells have been especially used in studies on CvME pathway. A study tested the endocytosis pathways involved in the transfection of PEI/DNA complexes with different cell lines. The result showed that in COS-7 cells, the clathrin-dependent pathway was the main contributor to the transfection process for both linear and branch PEIs [9]. Another study suggests that macropinosomes have a higher propensity to deliver PEI/DNA cargo than do endosomes in CHO and Hela cells [12]. Therefore, different cell lines involve different endocytic pathways, and cell type is the important factor that must be considered in such studies.

## 4. Tools for the study of uptake pathways

The study on the mechanisms of uptake pathways is important to the rational design of non-viral gene vectors because this step can determine the intracellular fate of complexes. However, because there are many factors that influence the pathway selection, how to conduct these studies is also a very complicated problem that needs to be discussed in detail.

Inhibitors are the effective tools to block specific pathway in order to determine whether it plays an important role in the uptake of complexes. However, none of the commonly used inhibitors of different uptake pathways is absolutely specific. All of them either affect the actin cytoskeleton with their side effects, or interfere with alternative uptake pathways simultaneously. In addition, they usually show cell type variations. The scope of the usage of commonly used inhibitors will be introduced according to the classification of uptake pathways in the following paragraphs of this section. The most direct way to distinguish endocytic pathways and non-endocytic pathways is to use the inhibitor or method of energy depletion, because most endocytic pathways are energy dependent. The commonly used inhibitors and methods are: low temperature (4 °C) and sodium azide (an ATPase inhibitor). Low temperature and ATP inhibitor should be used together in some conditions because some of the non-endocytic pathways are also sensitive to low temperature [42, 49].

To distinguish the phagocytic and macropinocytic pathways with CME and CvME pathways, the commonly used inhibitors and methods for phagocytic and macropinocytic pathways are: inhibitors of sodium-proton exchange "amiloride and its derivatives", F-actindepolymerizing drugs "cytochalasin D and latrunculins", inhibitors of phosphoinositide metabolism "wortmannin and LY290042", and protein kinase C activator "phorbol esters". Except phorbol esters, the specificity of all the inhibitors is still in doubt as depolymerizing F-actin and inhibition of phosphoinositide metabolism may also disrupt the other two endocytic pathways. For example, cytochalasin D is also used as the inhibitor for CvME [50]. Within these inhibitors, amiloride and its derivatives may be considered as the first choice for their fewest side effects. Rottlerin, a novel macropinocytosis inhibitor which is rapid acting, irreversible, and selective, was discovered in 2005. In 2009, Hufnagel et al. found that rottlerin can specifically inhibit the transfection efficiency of PEI (25 kDa)/DNA complexes on Hela and CHO-K1 cells up to 50%, which verified the important role of FPE in the non-viral gene delivery by PEI (25 kDa) [12].

The commonly used inhibitors and methods for clathrin-mediated endocytosis are: Hypertonic sucrose (0.4–0.5 M), potassium depletion, cytosolic acidification, chlorpromazine (50–

100 μM), monodansylcadaverine (MDC), phenylarsine oxide. However, all of them have been shown to be able to inhibit macropinocytosis, thus cannot be used to distinguish the clathrin-mediated endocytic pathway and the macropinocytic pathway. Besides this, all these inhibitors can influence the cortical actin cytoskeleton more or less, which can cause non-specific cytotoxicity. However, potassium depletion, chlorpromazine, and MDC are the relatively better choices than the other ones for the initial discrimination of clathrin-mediated endocytic pathway [51].

As to caveolae-mediated endocytic pathway, the commonly used inhibitors and methods are: statins, methyl-β-cyclodextrin (MβCD), filipin, nystatin, genestein, and cholesterol oxidase. Among them, the incubation with filipin, nystatin, and cholesterol oxidase produce the fewest side effects. The chronic inhibition of cholesterol synthesis by statins or acute cholesterol depletion by MβCD nonspecifically disrupts intracellular vesicle trafficking and the actin cytoskeleton. Also, the specificity of genestein is still in doubt for its nonspecific disruption of the actin network. That being so, appropriate controls should be included when filipin, nystatin, and cholesterol oxidase are used [51].

The inhibitors for the study of intracellular fates of complexes are also very important. Monensin, bafilomycin A can inhibit the acidification of endosomes, thus preventing their maturation and fusion into lysosomes [52, 53]. Chloroquine is another inhibitor that accumulates in endosomes/lysosomes and causes the swelling and disruption of endocytic vesicles by osmotic effects [21]. Last but not least, the cell-dependence of inhibitors should be noted when experiments are carried out. For example, chlorpromazine treatment inhibited the uptake of transferrin, a marker for CME by ~50% in D407 and HUH-7 cells. However, it showed no or little significant inhibitory capacity in ARPE-19 and Vero cells or even an enhanced effect in COS-7 cells [54, 55]. Therefore, a range of concentration with lowest cytotoxicity and sufficient inhibitory efficiency should be determined first when the inhibitor is used on the cell for the first time. Then, the lack of absolute specificity can be compensated by the combined application of biological methods such as siRNA silencing, transient or stable expression of dominant-negative proteins, and reconstruction of proteins by knockout mutants, all of which aremore specific than classical chemical inhibitors. For example, mutant dynamin has been successfully used to prove the necessity of dynamin in the endocytic pathways of transferrin receptors and EGF receptors [55]. A constitutive knockdown technique through RNAi has been used to prove the role of an essential accessory protein "epsin" in the CME pathway [56]. Another efficient way of making up the pitfalls of nonspecific inhibitors is the combined usage of fluorescently labeled gene complexes and fluorescent probes that are specifically internalized through certain uptake pathways.

Except for inhibitors, molecular probes and markers are also important tools for the study of uptake pathways for non-viral gene complexes. They can be used together with the classical chemical inhibitors or biological inhibitors to make the results more convincing. There are several classical molecular probes that are known to be specifically internalized through each uptake pathway. Transferrin is often used as a probe of CME pathway in many studies [12, 57, 58]. Transferrin receptor (TFR) mediates transferrin uptake by CME, so that it can be used as a CME marker and detected by anti-TFR [59].

Cholera toxin beta subunit (CTBs) is commonly used as a probe for CvME [12, 57]. However, Lisa et al. argued that CTBs binds receptors that are contained in lipid-rich areas and are internalized via a mechanism similar to CvME, because CTBs uptake is unaffected by a clathrin inhibitor and 33% uptake remains after treatment with a specific caveola inhibitor. Therefore, CTBs may enter into the cells via another unknown clathrin-independent mechanism [60]. In addition, caveolin-1 is also an important marker for CvME, as it is specifically involved in the formation of caveosome [29].

Dextran is the popular probe for macropinocytosis in some studies because it can accumulate in the endo-lysosome compartment [57]. As to phagocytosis, large (2 µm) microspheres are usually used as the probes. To solve the issue about the intracellular fate of complexes, a group of the specific markers or biological dyes are necessary to colocalize the non-viral gene complexes and intracellular organelles. TFR is used as a classical early endosome marker because it is transported into an early endosome when transferrin is internalized. EEA-1 is a hydrophilic peripheral membrane protein present in cytosol and membrane fractions. It colocalizes with TFR, and immunoelectron microscopy shows that it is associated with tubulovesicular early endosomes [61]. The lysosome-associated type 1 membrane glycoproteins LAMP-1 and LAMP-2 are localized primarily on the periphery of the lysosome, and can be used as markers for lysosome [62, 63]. The different roles of EEA-1 and LAMP in the endolysosome pathway allow us to know the stage in which the uptake carries on. Other endosome or lysosome markers are the Rab family proteins. They are small GTPases that control multiple membrane trafficking events in the cell, and there are at least 60 Rab genes in the human genome [64]. Inside the Rab family, Rab5 and Rab7 are the most studied Rab variants, in which Rab5 is found to be the marker for early endosomes as it in part controls the invagination at the plasma membrane, endosomal fusion, motility, and signaling [63], and Rab7 is found to be the marker for late endosomes and lysosomes as it controls the aggregation, fusion, and maintenance of perinuclear lysosome compartment [65].

| Pathways | inhibitors | markers |
|---|---|---|
| Phagocytosis | Amiloride, cytochalasin D, latrunculins, wortmannin, LY290042, sodium azide | Large microspheres (2 µm) |
| CME | Chlorpromazine, monodansylcadaverine, phenylarsine oxide, sodium azide | Transferrin, lactosylceramide, TFR |
| CvME | Filipin, nystatin, cholesterol oxidase, statins, genestein, MβCD, sodium azide | CTBs, caveolin-1 |
| Macropinocytosis | Rottlerin, amiloride, cytochalasin D, latrunculins, wortmannin, LY290042, sodium azide | Dextran |

**Table 2.** Inhibitors and markers

The organelle specific dyes are other ideal tools for the detection of colocalization, and they are relatively convenient. LysoTracker (red) and Lyso Sensor (green) are the widely used dyes for lysosomes. Cell light (red or green) are the widely used dyes for early endosomes. Combined with the confocal imaging technology, the colocalization of labeled non-viral gene complexes and intracellular compartments can be viewed intuitively. However, the classical confocal imaging technology can only provide the monolayer images, the information from which is not convincing enough. A novel three dimensionally integrated confocal technology is so strong that it can provide the intact information of a whole cell by scanning layer by layer.

# 5. Application of cellular uptake mechanism.

Based on the current understanding of cellular uptake mechanisms, one can rationally design vectors and improve their efficiency. Each pathway has advantages that need to be optimized and disadvantages that should be avoided (Table 3).

| Pathways | Advantages | Disadvantages |
|---|---|---|
| Phagocytosis | Specific cell-type targeting<br>Specific receptors | Lysosome involved<br>In vivo clearance |
| CME | Specific receptors | Lysosome involved |
| CvME | Bypass the lysosome<br>Specific receptors | Membrane structure dependent<br>Slower cellular uptaking |
| Macropinocytosis | Larger particles uptaking. | Non-specific |
| Non-endocytic | Bypass the lysosome | Non-specific |

**Table 3.** Characteristics of pathways.

## 5.1. Endo-lysosomal escape

Endo-lysosomal escape is one of the most crucial issues in non-viral vector design. Non-viral delivery systems, such as polyplexes and lipoplexes, will be trapped and degraded in the lysosomes if their cellular uptake pathways involve endo-lysosomes. As discussed above, some of the uptake pathways involve endo-lysosomes, such as CME and phagocytosis. CvME is known to bypass the endo-lysosomes. Similarly, macropinocytosis is known to not have any associations with endo-lysosomes [66, 67], but some studies have suggested that it involves lysosomes [67, 68]. These contradictory data may be dependent on cell type. Stimulating special pathway to bypass endo-lysosomes is a novel direction to improve efficiency. This will be discussed later.

A non-viral delivery system uptaken by endo-lysosomes dependent pathways must be capable of escaping endo-lysosomes. From early endosome to late endosome transport, a maturation process involving compartment acidification by proton pumps located on the endosomal membrane exists. Some non-viral vectors exhibit the ability to escape the endo-lysosome, called *proton sponge*, such as PEI [10, 69, 70]. PEI contains a nitrogen atom that can be protonated, and this serves to consume endosomal protons because endosomes acidify their microenvironment. As a result, an increase in endosomal chloride anion, which diffuses into the endosomes with the protons, leads to an increase in osmotic pressure, thus inducing osmotic swelling [69]. Therefore, the endosome might break down and release PEI. This mode of action has been widely incorporated in recent non-viral vector designs. However, a pDAMA-based vector with endosomal buffering capacity has been reported to show no endosomal escape activity in cell-based assay, indicating that the proton sponge hypothesis may not be applicable in some cases. These findings warrant further elucidation and investigation of the mechanism of non-viral gene delivery [71].

For lipoplexes, the cationic liposome can interact with the anionic cytoplasmic facing monolayer lipid of endosome and release the DNA from the endosome through the flip-flop mechanism [72]. 1,2-Dioleoylsn-glycero-3-phosphatidylethanolamine (DOPE), the pH-sensitive fusogenic lipid additive, is very helpful to the displacement of the anionic lipds from the cytoplasm-facingmonolayer of the endosomal membrane to the opposite direction via a flip-flop mechanism. However, the serum components are known to inactivate and destabilize the lipoplex structures that contain DOPE [73].

Viruses have the ability to destabilize the endosomal membrane, which explains why many proteins from different viruses are being used [69]. Some viruses are well known to use fusogenic peptides to cross the endosomal membrane and reach the cytosol [21]. The process by which viruses destabilize endosomal membranes in an acidification-dependent manner has been mimicked with synthetic peptides containing the amino-terminal 20-amino-acid sequence of the influenza virus HA [70]. Generally, short sequences of only 20 amino acids are needed for membrane destabilization, and they usually contain a high content of basic residues [74].

Cell-penetrating peptides (CPPs) are used to enhance endosomal escape. The HIV-1 Tat protein is the first CPP to be discovered. It transactivates the transcription of the HIV-1 genome, has been observed to cross the plasma membrane by itself, leading to the identification of a peptide fragment (49–59 amino acids) that confers cell permeability to the protein (Tat peptide), and is one of the better characterized CPPs [75]. Most of the CPPs contain a high density of basic amino acids (arginines and/orlysines), which are proposed to interact with the anionic surface of the plasma membrane and enhance internalization of the peptides [75]. These peptides adopt an a -helical structure at endosomal pH leading to hydrophobic and hydrophilic faces that can interact with the endosomal membrane to cause disruption and pore formation [74].

## 5.2. Optimization of CvME

CvME is considered an alternative pathway that can bypass the endo-lysosomes. As gene materials will not be degraded in the lysosomal compartments, we can take advantage of CvME to improve the efficiency of transfection. For example, Nathan P. et al. targeted complexes (PEI–DNA) in CvME and CME with folic acid and transferrin, respectively; however, only vectors via CvME successfully delivered genes, as CvME is avoidant of lysosomes.

These data demonstrate that the uptake mechanism and subsequent endocytic processing are important design parameters for gene delivery materials [76]. However, the key is controlling the uptake mechanism.

Particle size is a very important factor for uptake mechanisms. In a previous study, three particles (20, 40, and 100 nm) were investigated for their uptake efficiency via CvME in endothelial cells. The results showed that the uptake efficiency levels of the 20- and 40-nm nanoparticles were 5–10 times greater than that of the 100-nm particles [6], indicating that small particles can be uptaken by CvME more efficiently compared with large ones. However, another study found that the uptake of microspheres with a diameter <200 nm in non-phagocytic B16 cells involved CME. With increasing size, a shift to a mechanism that relied on a caveolae-mediated pathway became apparent, which became the predominant pathway of entry for particles measuring 500 nm in size [77]. This can be attributed to the fact that the mechanism of CvME is cell type dependent in some cases. According to the target cell type, the mechanism must be fully studied before designing a vector.

CvME is a kind of receptor-mediated endocytosis pathway. As a result, some specific ligands can mediate CvME via ligand–receptor binding. The insulin receptor [30], epidermal growth factor (EGF) receptor [31], transforming growth factor beta (TGFbeta) receptor [78] have been found to mediate this pathway. Another study used the cyclic Asn–Gly–Arg peptide to enhance gene transfection efficiency in CD13-positive vascular endothelial cells via CvME [79]. However, cyclic RGD ligands have been reported to facilitate CvME of thiolated c(RGDfK)-polyethylene glycol (PEG)-b-PLL micelles without high endosomal-disrupting properties and thus improve transfection efficiency [80]. The cyclic RGD peptide ligands c(RGDfK) can selectively recognize $\alpha v\beta 3$ and $\alpha v\beta 5$ integrin receptors on the cell surface. The receptors can mediate CvME and bypass endo-lysosomes. The $\alpha v\beta 3$ and $\alpha v\beta 5$ integrin receptors overexpressed on endothelial cells of tumor capillaries and neointimal tissues. As a result, the vectors with cyclic RGD peptide ligands can be used for cancer gene therapy.

Cellular stress can also be used to control the cellular uptake mechanism. Heat shock and hyperosmotic shock can stimulate caveolin internalization [81]. Recent research has shown that hypertonic exposure of alveolar cells caused down-regulation of CME and fluid-phase endocytosis while stimulating CvME. An osmotic polymannitol-based gene transporter that can increase caveolae-mediated endocytosis was designed taking advantage of this mechanism [82]. The possible mechanisms have been discussed. Non-penetrating osmolytes tend to draw water from the intracellular space through an osmotic gradient, cause cell hypertonic stress accompanied by cell shrinkage. Responding the cellular hypertonic stress, phosphorylation of caveolin-1 is mediated by Src-kinase. Src-kinase-mediated phosphorylation of caveolin-1 is required for caveolae budding. Finally the CvME is stimulated.

### 5.3. Inhibition of phagocytosis

After *in vivo* administration, the non-viral delivery system can be uptaken by macrophages and then cleared. This macrophage clearance effect mainly via phagocytosis is one of the main barriers for non-viral gene delivery. Numerous methods are used to avoid phagocytosis of macrophages in vector design. Antibodies are being widely used for targeting non-viral gene delivery. However, the constant fragments can be recognized by phagocytosis and then uptaken by macrophages. Therefore, antibodies that lack constant fragments are sometimes used to help non-viral vectors avoid recognition and clearance by macrophages *in vivo* [83].

Other vectors can also be recognized by macrophages. As discussed above, some cationic polyplexes or lipoplexes will be tagged by some opsonins and then recognized *in vivo*. PE-Gylation is widely used to avoid the *in vivo* clearance effect by phagocytosis. The highly hydrophilic nature of PEG produces a hydration shell around its conjugated partner, hence reducing intermolecular interactions and, consequently, toxicity [84]. As an effect of reducing intermolecular interactions, PEGylation can effectively avoid phagocytosis; moreover, *in vivo* studies have reported on long circulating half-life of PEGylated vectors [85].

However, some studies have shown that PEGylation can reduce the efficiency of vectors [84] possibly because PEGylation may inhibit cellular uptake and endosomal escape of the vectors. One study compared non-PEGylated and PEGylated liposomes, with the data showing that PEGylated liposomes have poor endosomal escape capability as non-PEGylated liposomes can escape from endosome efficiently [86]. The inhibitory effects of PEGylation depend on some factors. A study about PEGylated cationic liposomes demonstrated that acid-labile PEGylation liposomes have higher transfection efficiency than acid-stable PEGylation ones, which can be ascribed to the more efficient endosomal escape activity of acid-labile PEGylation liposomes [87]. The possible mechanism involved here is that the PEG of acid-labile PEGylation liposomes can be cleaved under low pH (endosomal compartments), allowing the vector to fully interact with the endosomal membrane. So other biodegradable shielding methods should be better than classical PEGylation. According to this hypothesis, recently, an alternative to PEGylation was designed. This work reports, for the first time, the use of hydroxyethyl starch (HES) for the controlled shielding/deshielding of polyplexes. Non-viral delivery systems can be protected by HES shielding, and the HES can then be degraded *in vivo*, indicating that HES shielding has less influence on the efficiency of vectors compared with PEGylation [88].

# 6. Conclusion

In summary, cellular uptake is the most important intracellular process. Understanding cellular uptake mechanisms is essential to determining the limits of gene delivery. Different pathways have different intracellular fates. Some vectors can enter cells via endo-lysosomal pathways. Thus, some methods have to be used to protect genes against degradation in lysosomes. Optimizing CvME can successfully deliver genes by avoiding endo-lysosomes. Each pathway has its own disadvantages, and learning how to inhibit certain pathways is significant in some cases. In conclusion, taking advantage of cellular uptake mechanisms and knowing how to control them hold considerable potential for improving the efficiency of gene delivery.

# Acknowledgements

This work was supported by grants from The Ministry of Science and Technology of China (No.2011DFA30790), National Natural Science Foundation of China (No. 81190133), Chinese Academy of Sciences (No.XDA01030404, KSCX2-EW-Q-1-07), Science and Technology Commission of Shanghai Municipality (No.11QH1401600), Shanghai Municipal Education Commission (No.10SG22).

# Author details

Shengnan Xiang and Xiaoling Zhang

*Address all correspondence to: xlzhang@sibs.ac.cn

The Key Laboratory of Stem Cell Biology, Institute of Health Sciences, Shanghai Jiao Tong University School of Medicine (SJTUSM) & Shanghai Institutes for Biological Sciences (SIBS), Chinese Academy of Sciences (CAS), Shanghai, China

# References

[1] Gao, K. and L. Huang, *Nonviral methods for siRNA delivery.* Mol Pharm, 2009. 6(3): p. 651-8.

[2] Luo, D. and W.M. Saltzman, *Synthetic DNA delivery systems.* Nat Biotechnol, 2000. 18(1): p. 33-7.

[3] Wiethoff, C.M. and C.R. Middaugh, *Barriers to nonviral gene delivery.* J Pharm Sci, 2003. 92(2): p. 203-17.

[4] Akinc, A., et al., *A combinatorial library of lipid-like materials for delivery of RNAi therapeutics.* Nat Biotechnol, 2008. 26(5): p. 561-9.

[5] Whitehead, K.A., R. Langer, and D.G. Anderson, *Knocking down barriers: advances in siRNA delivery.* Nat Rev Drug Discov, 2009. 8(2): p. 129-38.

[6] Wang, Z., et al., *Size and dynamics of caveolae studied using nanoparticles in living endothelial cells.* ACS Nano, 2009. 3(12): p. 4110-6.

[7] Harashima, H., Y. Shinohara, and H. Kiwada, *Intracellular control of gene trafficking using liposomes as drug carriers.* Eur J Pharm Sci, 2001. 13(1): p. 85-9.

[8] Boussif, O., et al., *A versatile vector for gene and oligonucleotide transfer into cells in culture and in vivo: polyethylenimine.* Proc Natl Acad Sci U S A, 1995. 92(16): p. 7297-301.

[9] von Gersdorff, K., et al., *The internalization route resulting in successful gene expression depends on both cell line and polyethylenimine polyplex type.* Mol Ther, 2006. 14(5): p. 745-53.

[10]  Rejman, J., A. Bragonzi, and M. Conese, *Role of clathrin- and caveolae-mediated endocytosis in gene transfer mediated by lipo- and polyplexes.* Mol Ther, 2005. 12(3): p. 468-74.

[11]  Hillaireau, H. and P. Couvreur, *Nanocarriers' entry into the cell: relevance to drug delivery.* Cell Mol Life Sci, 2009. 66(17): p. 2873-96.

[12]  Hufnagel, H., et al., *Fluid phase endocytosis contributes to transfection of DNA by PEI-25.* Mol Ther, 2009. 17(8): p. 1411-7.

[13]  Aderem, A. and D.M. Underhill, *Mechanisms of phagocytosis in macrophages.* Annu Rev Immunol, 1999. 17: p. 593-623.

[14]  Rabinovitch, M., *Professional and non-professional phagocytes: an introduction.* Trends Cell Biol, 1995. 5(3): p. 85-7.

[15]  Matsui, H., et al., *Loss of binding and entry of liposome-DNA complexes decreases transfection efficiency in differentiated airway epithelial cells.* J Biol Chem, 1997. 272(2): p. 1117-26.

[16]  Kopatz, I., J.S. Remy, and J.P. Behr, *A model for non-viral gene delivery: through syndecan adhesion molecules and powered by actin.* J Gene Med, 2004. 6(7): p. 769-76.

[17]  Vonarbourg, A., et al., *Parameters influencing the stealthiness of colloidal drug delivery systems.* Biomaterials, 2006. 27(24): p. 4356-73.

[18]  Wattendorf, U., et al., *Mannose-based molecular patterns on stealth microspheres for receptor-specific targeting of human antigen-presenting cells.* Langmuir, 2008. 24(20): p. 11790-802.

[19]  Chaudhuri, G., *Scavenger receptor-mediated delivery of antisense mini-exon phosphorothioate oligonucleotide to Leishmania-infected macrophages. Selective and efficient elimination of the parasite.* Biochem Pharmacol, 1997. 53(3): p. 385-91.

[20]  Areschoug, T. and S. Gordon, *Scavenger receptors: role in innate immunity and microbial pathogenesis.* Cell Microbiol, 2009. 11(8): p. 1160-9.

[21]  Wattiaux, R., et al., *Endosomes, lysosomes: their implication in gene transfer.* Adv Drug Deliv Rev, 2000. 41(2): p. 201-8.

[22]  Pearse, B.M., *Clathrin: a unique protein associated with intracellular transfer of membrane by coated vesicles.* Proc Natl Acad Sci U S A, 1976. 73(4): p. 1255-9.

[23]  Rappoport, J.Z., *Focusing on clathrin-mediated endocytosis.* Biochem J, 2008. 412(3): p. 415-23.

[24]  Schmid, S.L., *Clathrin-coated vesicle formation and protein sorting: an integrated process.* Annu Rev Biochem, 1997. 66: p. 511-48.

[25]  Brodsky, F.M., et al., *Biological basket weaving: formation and function of clathrin-coated vesicles.* Annu Rev Cell Dev Biol, 2001. 17: p. 517-68.

[26]  Sakaguchi, N., et al., *Effect of transferrin as a ligand of pH-sensitive fusogenic liposome-lipoplex hybrid complexes.* Bioconjug Chem, 2008. 19(8): p. 1588-95.

[27]  Takei, K. and V. Haucke, *Clathrin-mediated endocytosis: membrane factors pull the trigger.* Trends Cell Biol, 2001. 11(9): p. 385-91.

[28]  van der Aa, M.A., et al., *Cellular uptake of cationic polymer-DNA complexes via caveolae plays a pivotal role in gene transfection in COS-7 cells.* Pharm Res, 2007. 24(8): p. 1590-8.

[29]  Nichols, B., *Caveosomes and endocytosis of lipid rafts.* J Cell Sci, 2003. 116(Pt 23): p. 4707-14.

[30]  Fagerholm, S., et al., *Rapid insulin-dependent endocytosis of the insulin receptor by caveolae in primary adipocytes.* PLoS One, 2009. 4(6): p. e5985.

[31]  Ning, Y., T. Buranda, and L.G. Hudson, *Activated epidermal growth factor receptor induces integrin alpha2 internalization via caveolae/raft-dependent endocytic pathway.* J Biol Chem, 2007. 282(9): p. 6380-7.

[32]  Escriche, M., et al., *Ligand-induced caveolae-mediated internalization of A1 adenosine receptors: morphological evidence of endosomal sorting and receptor recycling.* Exp Cell Res, 2003. 285(1): p. 72-90.

[33]  Sarkar, K., et al., *Selective inhibition by rottlerin of macropinocytosis in monocyte-derived dendritic cells.* Immunology, 2005. 116(4): p. 513-24.

[34]  Haigler, H.T., J.A. McKanna, and S. Cohen, *Rapid stimulation of pinocytosis in human carcinoma cells A-431 by epidermal growth factor.* J Cell Biol, 1979. 83(1): p. 82-90.

[35]  Racoosin, E.L. and J.A. Swanson, *Macrophage colony-stimulating factor (rM-CSF) stimulates pinocytosis in bone marrow-derived macrophages.* J Exp Med, 1989. 170(5): p. 1635-48.

[36]  Swanson, J.A., *Phorbol esters stimulate macropinocytosis and solute flow through macrophages.* J Cell Sci, 1989. 94 ( Pt 1): p. 135-42.

[37]  Norbury, C.C., et al., *Constitutive macropinocytosis allows TAP-dependent major histocompatibility complex class I presentation of exogenous soluble antigen by bone marrow-derived dendritic cells.* Eur J Immunol, 1997. 27(1): p. 280-8.

[38]  Hewlett, L.J., A.R. Prescott, and C. Watts, *The coated pit and macropinocytic pathways serve distinct endosome populations.* J Cell Biol, 1994. 124(5): p. 689-703.

[39]  Swanson, J.A. and C. Watts, *Macropinocytosis.* Trends Cell Biol, 1995. 5(11): p. 424-8.

[40]  Jones, A.T., *Macropinocytosis: searching for an endocytic identity and role in the uptake of cell penetrating peptides.* J Cell Mol Med, 2007. 11(4): p. 670-84.

[41]  Gupta, B., T.S. Levchenko, and V.P. Torchilin, *Intracellular delivery of large molecules and small particles by cell-penetrating proteins and peptides.* Adv Drug Deliv Rev, 2005. 57(4): p. 637-51.

[42]  Hong, S., et al., *Interaction of poly(amidoamine) dendrimers with supported lipid bilayers and cells: hole formation and the relation to transport.* Bioconjug Chem, 2004. 15(4): p. 774-82.

[43]  Lee, H., I.K. Kim, and T.G. Park, *Intracellular trafficking and unpacking of siRNA/quantum dot-PEI complexes modified with and without cell penetrating peptide: confocal and flow cytometric FRET analysis.* Bioconjug Chem, 2010. 21(2): p. 289-95.

[44]  Zuhorn, I.S., R. Kalicharan, and D. Hoekstra, *Lipoplex-mediated transfection of mammalian cells occurs through the cholesterol-dependent clathrin-mediated pathway of endocytosis.* J Biol Chem, 2002. 277(20): p. 18021-8.

[45]  Zhang, Y., et al., *A novel PEGylation of chitosan nanoparticles for gene delivery.* Biotechnol Appl Biochem, 2007. 46(Pt 4): p. 197-204.

[46]  Chithrani, B.D., A.A. Ghazani, and W.C. Chan, *Determining the size and shape dependence of gold nanoparticle uptake into mammalian cells.* Nano Lett, 2006. 6(4): p. 662-8.

[47]  Chithrani, B.D. and W.C. Chan, *Elucidating the mechanism of cellular uptake and removal of protein-coated gold nanoparticles of different sizes and shapes.* Nano Lett, 2007. 7(6): p. 1542-50.

[48]  Koping-Hoggard, M., et al., *Relationship between the physical shape and the efficiency of oligomeric chitosan as a gene delivery system in vitro and in vivo.* J Gene Med, 2003. 5(2): p. 130-41.

[49]  Hong, S., et al., *The role of ganglioside GM1 in cellular internalization mechanisms of poly(amidoamine) dendrimers.* Bioconjug Chem, 2009. 20(8): p. 1503-13.

[50]  Parton, R.G., B. Joggerst, and K. Simons, *Regulated internalization of caveolae.* J Cell Biol, 1994. 127(5): p. 1199-215.

[51]  Ivanov, A.I., *Pharmacological inhibition of endocytic pathways: is it specific enough to be useful?* Methods Mol Biol, 2008. 440: p. 15-33.

[52]  Tartakoff, A.M., *Perturbation of vesicular traffic with the carboxylic ionophore monensin.* Cell, 1983. 32(4): p. 1026-8.

[53]  Drose, S. and K. Altendorf, *Bafilomycins and concanamycins as inhibitors of V-ATPases and P-ATPases.* J Exp Biol, 1997. 200(Pt 1): p. 1-8.

[54]  Vercauteren, D., et al., *The use of inhibitors to study endocytic pathways of gene carriers: optimization and pitfalls.* Mol Ther, 2010. 18(3): p. 561-9.

[55]  Damke, H., et al., *Induction of mutant dynamin specifically blocks endocytic coated vesicle formation.* J Cell Biol, 1994. 127(4): p. 915-34.

[56]  Vanden Broeck, D. and M.J. De Wolf, *Selective blocking of clathrin-mediated endocytosis by RNA interference: epsin as target protein.* Biotechniques, 2006. 41(4): p. 475-84.

[57]  Duchardt, F., et al., *A comprehensive model for the cellular uptake of cationic cell-penetrating peptides.* Traffic, 2007. 8(7): p. 848-66.

[58]  Alam, M.R., et al., *Intracellular delivery of an anionic antisense oligonucleotide via receptor-mediated endocytosis.* Nucleic Acids Res, 2008. 36(8): p. 2764-76.

[59]  Luhmann, T., et al., *Cellular uptake and intracellular pathways of PLL-g-PEG-DNA nanoparticles.* Bioconjug Chem, 2008. 19(9): p. 1907-16.

[60]  Bareford, L.M. and P.W. Swaan, *Endocytic mechanisms for targeted drug delivery*. Adv Drug Deliv Rev, 2007. 59(8): p. 748-58.

[61]  Mu, F.T., et al., *EEA1, an early endosome-associated protein. EEA1 is a conserved alpha-helical peripheral membrane protein flanked by cysteine "fingers" and contains a calmodulin-binding IQ motif*. J Biol Chem, 1995. 270(22): p. 13503-11.

[62]  Furuta, K., et al., *Differential expression of the lysosome-associated membrane proteins in normal human tissues*. Arch Biochem Biophys, 1999. 365(1): p. 75-82.

[63]  Duclos, S., R. Corsini, and M. Desjardins, *Remodeling of endosomes during lysosome biogenesis involves 'kiss and run' fusion events regulated by rab5*. J Cell Sci, 2003. 116(Pt 5): p. 907-18.

[64]  Stenmark, H. and V.M. Olkkonen, *The Rab GTPase family*. Genome Biol, 2001. 2(5): p. REVIEWS3007.

[65]  Bucci, C., et al., *Rab7: a key to lysosome biogenesis*. Mol Biol Cell, 2000. 11(2): p. 467-80.

[66]  Zhang, X.X., P.G. Allen, and M. Grinstaff, *Macropinocytosis is the major pathway responsible for DNA transfection in CHO cells by a charge-reversal amphiphile*. Mol Pharm, 2011. 8(3): p. 758-66.

[67]  Falcone, S., et al., *Macropinocytosis: regulated coordination of endocytic and exocytic membrane traffic events*. J Cell Sci, 2006. 119(Pt 22): p. 4758-69.

[68]  Racoosin, E.L. and J.A. Swanson, *Macropinosome maturation and fusion with tubular lysosomes in macrophages*. J Cell Biol, 1993. 121(5): p. 1011-20.

[69]  Kamiya, H., et al., *Intracellular trafficking and transgene expression of viral and non-viral gene vectors*. Adv Drug Deliv Rev, 2001. 52(3): p. 153-64.

[70]  Tseng, Y.C., S. Mozumdar, and L. Huang, *Lipid-based systemic delivery of siRNA*. Adv Drug Deliv Rev, 2009. 61(9): p. 721-31.

[71]  Funhoff, A.M., et al., *Endosomal escape of polymeric gene delivery complexes is not always enhanced by polymers buffering at low pH*. Biomacromolecules, 2004. 5(1): p. 32-9.

[72]  Zelphati, O. and F.C. Szoka, Jr., *Mechanism of oligonucleotide release from cationic liposomes*. Proc Natl Acad Sci U S A, 1996. 93(21): p. 11493-8.

[73]  Sakurai, F., et al., *Effects of erythrocytes and serum proteins on lung accumulation of lipoplexes containing cholesterol or DOPE as a helper lipid in the single-pass rat lung perfusion system*. Eur J Pharm Biopharm, 2001. 52(2): p. 165-72.

[74]  Martin, M.E. and K.G. Rice, *Peptide-guided gene delivery*. AAPS J, 2007. 9(1): p. E18-29.

[75]  Endoh, T. and T. Ohtsuki, *Cellular siRNA delivery using cell-penetrating peptides modified for endosomal escape*. Adv Drug Deliv Rev, 2009. 61(9): p. 704-9.

[76]  Gabrielson, N.P. and D.W. Pack, *Efficient polyethylenimine-mediated gene delivery proceeds via a caveolar pathway in HeLa cells*. J Control Release, 2009. 136(1): p. 54-61.

[77]  Rejman, J., et al., *Size-dependent internalization of particles via the pathways of clathrin- and caveolae-mediated endocytosis*. Biochem J, 2004. 377(Pt 1): p. 159-69.

[78] Razani, B., et al., *Caveolin-1 regulates transforming growth factor (TGF)-beta/SMAD signaling through an interaction with the TGF-beta type I receptor.* J Biol Chem, 2001. 276(9): p. 6727-38.

[79] Liu, C., et al., *Enhanced gene transfection efficiency in CD13-positive vascular endothelial cells with targeted poly(lactic acid)-poly(ethylene glycol) nanoparticles through caveolae-mediated endocytosis.* J Control Release, 2011. 151(2): p. 162-75.

[80] Oba, M., et al., *Polyplex micelles with cyclic RGD peptide ligands and disulfide cross-links directing to the enhanced transfection via controlled intracellular trafficking.* Mol Pharm, 2008. 5(6): p. 1080-92.

[81] Kang, Y.S., Y.G. Ko, and J.S. Seo, *Caveolin internalization by heat shock or hyperosmotic shock.* Exp Cell Res, 2000. 255(2): p. 221-8.

[82] Park, T.E., et al., *Selective stimulation of caveolae-mediated endocytosis by an osmotic poly-mannitol-based gene transporter.* Biomaterials, 2012. 33(29): p. 7272-81.

[83] Ikeda, Y. and K. Taira, *Ligand-targeted delivery of therapeutic siRNA.* Pharm Res, 2006. 23(8): p. 1631-40.

[84] Fitzsimmons, R.E. and H. Uludag, *Specific effects of PEGylation on gene delivery efficacy of polyethylenimine: Interplay between PEG substitution and N/P ratio.* Acta Biomater, 2012.

[85] Chaudhari, K.R., et al., *Opsonization, biodistribution, cellular uptake and apoptosis study of PEGylated PBCA nanoparticle as potential drug delivery carrier.* Pharm Res, 2012. 29(1): p. 53-68.

[86] Remaut, K., et al., *Pegylation of liposomes favours the endosomal degradation of the delivered phosphodiester oligonucleotides.* J Control Release, 2007. 117(2): p. 256-66.

[87] Chan, C.L., et al., *Endosomal escape and transfection efficiency of PEGylated cationic liposome-DNA complexes prepared with an acid-labile PEG-lipid.* Biomaterials, 2012. 33(19): p. 4928-35.

[88] Noga, M., et al., *Controlled shielding and deshielding of gene delivery polyplexes using hydroxyethyl starch (HES) and alpha-amylase.* J Control Release, 2012. 159(1): p. 92-103.

# Chapter 7

# Polylipid Nanoparticle,
# a Novel Lipid-Based Vector for Liver Gene Transfer

Yahan Fan and Jian Wu

Additional information is available at the end of the chapter

## 1. Introduction

Lipid nanoparticles (LNP) are invaluable carriers for drug and gene delivery, and they are classified as cationic, neutral and anionic depending on the electronic charges existing on the surface of the vesicles [1]. These charges are originated from the charged lipids from which lipid nanoparticles are formulated. Cationic LNP are commonly used for DNA or RNA carriers due to their interaction with negatively-charged nucleotide. Both neutral and negatively-charged LNPs are used for drug delivery [2] and may be formulated as sterically stable LNPs (SSLNPs), which are amendable for cell type-specific or tissue-specific targeting delivery [3]. For liver drug delivery, tremendous efforts have been made to develop cell type-selective lipid-based drug carriers. Effective approaches in targeting hepatocytes, Kupffer cells and hepatic stellate cells have been evaluated in small animals [3, 4], and some of them may be translational to clinical application [5]. These approaches are referable when cationic LNPs are considered for cell type-selective gene delivery. A prerequisite for the success of gene therapy for liver disorders is the development of powerful gene carriers. Non-viral vectors have been very successful for gene transfer in an *in vitro* setting, in terms of efficiency of lipofection, applicability in variety of cell types, and amending ability of cell type-specific delivery (Fig. 1). The clinical application of LNP-mediated gene transfer has been hampered by low efficiency, instability in the bloodstream, short-term transgene expression and toxicity. These shortcomings are the bottle neck hindering the gene transfer employing LNPs as carriers for delivery of function gene(s) to solid organs, and are the challenges in moving from small to large animals of potential gene carriers and approaches, and in the translation to clinical application. However, the polylipid nanoparticles (PLNP) we have developed over the past decade represent one of the few formulations that are applicable for *in vivo* gene transfer [6], due to a high DNA-packaging capacity, an extremely low binding rate to serum proteins, low toxicity, and amendable synthetic approaches [7, 8]. This chapter intends to introduce the characteristics of this formulation, and to discuss our efforts in moving the non-viral gene transfer platform from small to large animals towards clinical applications.

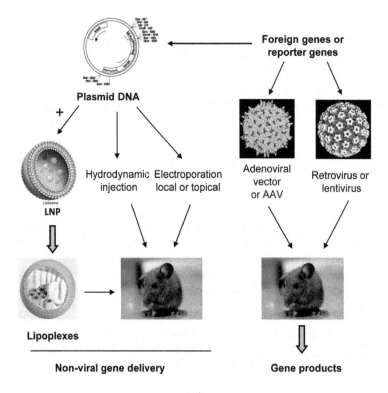

**Figure 1.** *In vivo* **gene transfer mediated by viral or non-viral vectors.** Viral vectors, such as lentiviral or retroviral vectors, which lead to integration of transgene in the host genome, give rise to long-term transgene expression. However, they may cause insertion-induced mutation that is oncogenic. Adenoviral or adeno-associated viral (AAV) vectors often yield a high level of transgene expression in host organs. However, generation of antibodies against viral components is still a concern. Non-viral gene transfer may be achieved by direct plasmid administration with local electroporation or a hydrodynamic approach. The latter is only applicable in mice. Lipid nanoparticle (LNP)-mediated gene transfer becomes a useful approach which is often very successful for *in vitro* gene transfer. Few formulations of cationic LNPs are valuable for *in vivo* gene transfer. There has been a still demand in improving their *in vivo* stability and gene transfer efficacy.

There are a number of critical components for a potential gene therapy product to move from one step to the next in this pipeline. Promisingly, LNP-mediated gene transfection for the treatment of genetic and metabolic disorders or tumors has been moved to clinical trial phases (http://clinicaltrials.gov). A phase I pilot study of gene therapy for cystic fibrosis using cationic liposome-mediated gene transfer (NCT00004471) has been completed. A phase I trial of intratumoral epidermal growth factor receptor (EGFR) antisense DNA delivered by DC-Chol liposomes in advanced head and neck cancer, including oral squamous cell carcinoma (NCT00009841) and DOTAP-Chol-Fus1 liposome-mediated gene therapy for non-small cell lung cancer (NCT00059605] [9] were conducted respectively by University of Pittsburg and MD Anderson Cancer Center in collaboration with the National Cancer Institute (NCI). Fus1 is a tumor suppressive gene that has been shown to be effective in suppressing the growth of original or metastatic lesions of non-small lung cancer when it is delivered locally or systemically [10]. Thus, it appears that genetic therapy using LNPs as gene carriers has the potential to be specially tailored for genetic disorders or cancers.

## 2. Nanoparticle carriers for drug or gene delivery

Lipid-based gene carriers include liposomes (cationic or anionic), polymer and dendrimer nanoparticles. Cationic liposomes are capable of delivering genes to cells or tissues, and achieving maximal therapeutic efficiency with minimal adverse effects [1]. However, the use of cationic LNPs for *in vivo* DNA transfection is hindered by substantial problems; i.e. after intravenous administration, cationic LNPs bind to plasma protein and blood cells due to charge reaction. The resulting aggregates of carriers with proteins or cells block microcirculation or may be cleared rapidly [11, 12]. The common formulations for *in vivo* gene delivery are DOTMA or DOTAP-DOPE or DOTAP-cholesterol (Chol). These formulations are highly serum-reactive [6, 13]. Lungs are the major organ shown to be highly transfected probably due to the accumulation of aggregates of lipoplexes with serum proteins or blood cells when the lipoplexes are administrated intravenously [14]. For this reason, cationic LNPs were once used widely for gene delivery to the lungs; and later for treating lung cancers and metastasis with further optimization [10, 15, 16]. LNP-mediated gene delivery to the liver is more difficult than to lungs. For the development of the gene carriers, cationic LNP formulations, such as DC-Chol, DOTAP-Chol, are available for delivering genes to various tissues [17]. A few LNP formulations targeting hepatocellular carcinoma (HCC) have been developed for improving efficacies of drug therapy [18, 19]. In order to avoid the rapid clearance by the reticuloendothelial system (RES) and to increase the drug delivery through the enhanced permeability and retention (EPR) effect to a tumor site by passive targeting, novel strategies, such as reducing particle size, minimizing rigidity of lipids, generating amphiphilic vesicles and shielding from the recognition by RES system, have been attempted in formulating lipid-based drug/gene carriers [1, 2]. To reduce lysosomal degradation, pH-sensitive LNPs are prepared for drug or gene delivery [20]. These approaches may be instructive in the development of LNPs for gene transfer at different stages of preclinical translation.

Polymeric non-viral vectors have exhibited additional advantages of lower toxicity and immunogenicity [21, 22]. These vectors may offer the possibility of industrial production following good manufacturing practice (GMP). Amphiphilic polyethylene glycol (PEG) has been engineered as a linker, most for coupling peptides to cationic lipids. Other polymers, such as dendritic poly(L-lysine)-b-poly(L-lactide)-b-dendritic vector [23], poly (ethylenei-mine) (PEI) [24], poly (methacrylate) [25] and polyamidoamine dendrimers [26], have been demonstrated to be effective for *in vitro* gene delivery. However, striking issues still exist for cationic polymers regarding whether they are applicable for *in vivo* gene transfer to solid or-gans such as the liver, without significant adverse effects.

## 3. Liver-specific gene delivery

Because of our interest in gene therapy of liver disorders, we have focused our efforts on improving liver-based gene delivery. The pathogenesis of liver injury and fibrosis in-volves complicated interactions among different cell populations in the liver, soluble fac-tors, such as cytokines and reactive oxygen species (ROS), and the extracellular matrix components. In order to improve the efficacy in preventing hepatocellular injury, the use of LNPs that are capable of delivering hepatoprotective agents to the liver, selectively to hepatocytes, will increase local concentration of therapeutic agents, reduce adverse effects, and achieve maximal therapeutic efficiency. The parenchymal cell type in the liver is hep-atocytes, which are responsible for an array of metabolic function in the body and are of-ten damaged in a variety of pathological processes. The asialoglycoprotein receptor (ASGP-R) on mammalian hepatocytes provides a unique means for the development of liver-specific drug or gene carriers. The abundant receptors on hepatocytes specifically recognize the natural ligands, lectin and asialofetuin (AF), as well as those with terminal galactose or N-acetylgalactosamine residues, and hepatocytes endocytose these ligands for an intracellular degradation process [27, 28]. The use of its natural or synthetic ligands, such as galactosylated cholesterol, glycolipids or galactosylated polymers to label LNPs has achieved significant targeting efficacy to the liver [4, 28]. AF-labeled LNPs have been used for improving liver-targeting gene transfer in small animals [29], yet there have not been successful reports available in the translation to large animals, such as pigs [30]. In-stead, plasmid DNA was directly administrated into the hepatic vein through a catheter with a balloon closure of hepatic vein blood flow [30]. One particular attention has been drawn in terms of the use of AF-labeled drug carriers for HCC targeting. The expression of ASGP-R in HCC cells varies depending on the differentiation status of HCC cells [31]. In general, well-differentiated HCC usually expresses relatively high levels of hepatocyte-specific genes, including ASGP-R; whereas poorly-differentiated HCC expresses minimal or no hepatocyte-specific genes, including ASGP-R [32]. In most cases, there exists the dra-matic heterogeneity of liver-specific gene expression in human HCC tissues [33], and de-creased expression of ASGP-R was observed in liver cancer tissue [34]. Therefore, using AF or other galactosylated or lactosylated residues to label LNPs for drug or gene deliv-ery may not always be effective for patients with HCC, because HCC develops on a varie-ty of disease backgrounds and there is a striking variation in ASGP-R expression levels in HCC from different patients. Using well-differentiated hepatoma cells, such as HepG2, Hep3B and Huh-7 cells, as an *in vitro* screening tool may not necessarily reflect targeting efficacy to tumor-specific distribution *in vivo* [35].

High density lipoprotein (HDL) has a high drug carry capacity, and can be recognized by HDL receptors on hepatocytes. Recombinant HDL was utilized to deliver an anti-HBV peptide (nosiheptide) to the liver, and it was shown to achieve a selective distribution in hepatoma cells *in vitro* and a preferential liver distribution in rats [36]. Apolipoprotein E is cleared by hepatocytes, and it has been employed to be carriers for small interfering RNA (siRNA) delivery to hepatocytes [37].

Given the fact that hepatic stellate cells (HSCs) are the major cell type responsible for hepatic fibrosis, a repairing process that causes excess production of extracellular matrix components and deposition of fibrotic scaring in chronically injured liver [38], much attention has been focused on targeting this cell type in the last decade. A couple of cell surface molecules that are overexpressed on activated HSCs during hepatic fibrogenesis, such as insulin growth factor receptor II [39], collagen type VI and platelet-derived growth factor (PDGF) receptor β-subunit [40] are selected as the cell surface targets. Drug carriers labeled with specific peptides recognizing these cell surface molecules, such as cyclic peptide containing arginine-glycine-aspartate (RGD)-labeled sterical lipid nanoparticles [3] or Mannose-6-phosphate human serum albumin (M6P/HAS) [41] exhibited HSC-selective distribution. The RGD cyclic peptide was recently used as a targeting molecule for the recognition of activated HSCs in two animal models for early diagnosis of hepatic fibrosis with a SPECT imaging modality [42]. Using the retinol binding protein (RBP) in activated HSCs seems to be very effective in delivering siRNA against gp46 (rat homolog of human heat shock protein 47), and inhibiting fibrosis in two animal models [43].

Targeting approaches for drug or gene delivery to other non-parenchymal cell types, such as Kupffer cells or sinusoidal endothelial cells, are summarized recently [27]. These approaches are crucial in delivering agents which are anti-inflammatory or anti-oxidants to these cell types due to the fact that Kupffer cells are pivotal in the mediation of inflammatory responses and subsequent fibrogenesis [44].

## 4. Polylipid nanoparticle-mediated liver gene delivery

Compared to drug delivery, LNP-mediated *in vivo* gene delivery is still in its development stage; and many issues that affect delivery approaches and efficacy remain to be solved. The main issues include: 1) the formation of aggregates between cationic lipids and serum proteins bearing negative charges; 2) the administration routes of LNP-DNA complexes (lipoplexes); 3) intracellular trafficking from the cytoplasm to the nucleus; 4) the proliferative state of cells to be transfected; and 5) transient transgene expression for a short duration [6, 45]. Substantial efforts have been made to address these issues in our previous studies and by others [8, 46, 47]. Particularly, we polymerized an acrylamide lipid to generate a polycationic lipid (PCL), which was able to interact with plasmid DNA effectively and form compacted complexes as demonstrated by Raman microspectral analysis [8]. PCL has a unique molecular configuration and molecular weight distribution as indicated by mass spectrophotometrical analysis [8]. Moreover, this lipid can be synthesized in a multiple gram quantity in a laboratory, and the synthetic approach is amendable for industrial production at a quantity sufficient enough for large animal use [8]. PLNP was formulated with a neutral lipid, cholesterol. The PLNP size was reduced to approximately 100 nm in diameter [7], and the Zeta potential of PLNP was decreased to neutral by neutralizing extra-positive charges with excess plasmid DNA [8]. Not only was this formulation of PLNP non-toxic, but it also displayed transfection efficiency equivalent to other commercially available transfection agents, such as Lipofectamine in hepatoma cell lines [7]. Moreover, high-resolution fluorescent deconvolution microscopy documented that PLNP-mediated gene transfection led to earlier GFP expression in hepatoma cells than Lipofectamine [8]. The unique feature of this formulation is that it is extremely serum-resistant, and exposure to cell culture medium containing 50% fetal bovine serum for 24 hours did not affect its size significantly. PLNP reacted up to 30-fold less with serum proteins or blood cells after intravenous administration in comparison with DOTAP-DOPE or DOTAP-Chol formulations [6]. This feature makes PLNP formulation particularly useful for *in vivo* gene transfer. In the subsequent studies, we have proved that it is very effective in the transfer of reporter genes or function genes to normal mouse livers as demonstrated in Fig. 2 by bioluminescent imaging of firefly luciferase gene expression 24 hours after portal vein injection of PLNP-plasmid DNA complexes (polyplexes) or preclinical models [48, 49].

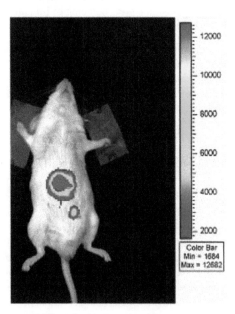

**Figure 2. PLNP-mediated gene transfer into mice through portal vein injection.** One day after the intravenous injection of polyplexes with pNDLux.2 plasmid encoding the firefly luciferase gene, the animal was imaged by CCD camera. The expression of luciferase was clearly shown in the liver area, demonstrating the effectiveness of this delivery approach and the applicability of a non-invasive imaging modality in the determination of transgene expression in animals.

We also developed an approach to promote normal hepatocytes to proliferate *in situ* without partial hepatectomy, which favors the transgene expression by lipofection but is not acceptable for clinical application [6]. Furthermore, placing an indwelling catheter in the portal vein allows repeated administration of polyplexes for sustained transgene expression [6]. All these efforts render our formulation of PLNP distinct from other lipid-based nanoparticles. Our animal experiments have clearly demonstrated that PLNP is characterized as extremely stable in the bloodstream, and highly effective in liver-based gene transfer when polyplexes are administrated through the portal vein [6, 17]. In comparison with other commonly used lipid formulations of nanoparticles, our formulation possesses the notable advantages essential for *in vivo* gene delivery as illustrated in Table 1.

| Characteristics | PCL | PLNP | Lipofectamine | DOTAP-Chol |
|---|---|---|---|---|
| Cationic lipid | Yes | LNP | LNP | LNP |
| Particle size (nm) | Irrelevant | 125±54 | 358 ±85 | 110±20 |
| Size changes(50%FBS) | Irrelevant | 100±20nm | 2206 ± 311 nm | 1050±100 nm |
| *In vitro* transfection efficiency Luciferase activity (in RLU) | Irrelevant | >10E7 | >10E7 | >10E7 |
| Cytotoxicity (LDH release) | Low or none | Normal | 10±3% (>5%) | 11±3.5% (>5%) |
| Binding rate to serum protein | Low | Low | Obvious | 20-30-fold higher than PLNP |
| *In vivo* stability | Irrelevant | Stable | Not determined | Instability |
| Usage | Raw material for PLNP | *In vitro* or *in vivo* transfection | *In vitro* transfection | *In vivo* transfection |

The content in this table was summarized according to our previous publications [6-8]. FBS = fetal bovine serum. RLU = relative light unit. LDH = lactate dehydrogenase.

**Table 1.** Comparison of common transfection agents for *in vitro* and *in vivo* application

# 5. Preclinical trials for proof of the concept

In order to demonstrate that our PLNP formulation is effective in delivering functional genes to the liver, we established a liver injury model in mice caused by the treatment with D-galactosamine (D-Gal) and lipopolysaccharide (LPS). This combination of D-Gal/LPS treatment resulted in a profound acute liver injury characterized by massive liver cell death through apoptosis, elevation of serum alanine aminotransferase (ALT), significant oxidant stress, depletion of the reduced form of glutathione and enhanced lipid peroxidation [50]. In

separate studies we have demonstrated that anti-oxidant enzyme such as extracellular superoxide dismutase (EC-SOD), SOD mimetics (MnTBAP) and catalase are effective in the
prevention of hepatic toxicity caused by xenobiotics in primary hepatocytes or hepatoma
cells [51-53], and they improved recipient survival and graft function and growth after
small-for-size liver transplantation in rats [54]. Therefore, we chose the human EC-SOD
gene as a functional gene to prove the feasibility. The EC-SOD gene product was exclusively
secreted into the extracellular space and functions as an ROS scavenger. ROS are generated
in both intracellular and extracellular spaces, and superoxide anions and hydrogen peroxide
($H_2O_2$) are able to cross the plasmatic membrane to enter the extracellular space [17]. It was
found that two days after portal vein injection of EC-SOD polyplexes, liver EC-SOD gene
expression was increased approximately 50-fold compared to the group receiving injection
of control plasmid polyplexes, and serum SOD activity was increased accordingly. On the
other hand, serum ALT was reduced to nearly one third in mice receiving EC-SOD polyplex
injection compared to those with D-Gal/LPS challenge, along with improved liver histology,
restored glutathione levels and decreased lipid peroxidation [48]. The findings of this preclinical trial confirmed the effectiveness of PLNP-mediated EC-SOD gene delivery to the liver, and that the delivery protected the mice from oxidant stress-associated liver injury. The
results also indicate that this anti-oxidant gene delivery approach could be useful in attenuating xenobiotics or drug metabolite-induced toxicity to the liver.

Ischemia/reperfusion (I/R)-associated donor organ damage is inevitable in all solid organ
transplantation, and is caused by enhanced oxidant stress with release of inflammatory
cytokines, such as tumor growth factor-$\alpha$ (TNF-$\alpha$) and interleukin 2 (IL-2). Although the
precise molecular mechanism of the I/R-associated liver injury remains to be investigated,
enhanced oxidant stress with release of superoxide anions or $H_2O_2$, depletion of the reduced form of glutathione and increased lipid peroxidation has been the key element in
the pathogenesis in orthotopic liver transplantation (OLT) or small size liver graft transplantation (SSLGT) [54-56]. Thus, it is rational to use of antioxidant gene transfer to mini-
mize oxidant stress and improve the donor organ quality and function after the
implantation. We delivered either EC-SOD, catalase gene or in combination, using the
same approach as described above. Two days after the delivery, the transgene expression
was increased for 10-50-fold, with increased SOD or catalase activity in the mouse liver.
This delivery led to a marked decrease in superoxide anion levels and $H_2O_2$ release along
with a decrease in serum ALT levels, liver lipid peroxidation and dramatic improvement
of liver histology [49]. This study was positively commented by two well-known hepatol-
ogists from Europe as an editorial, quoting "beyond a proof of the principle, the study
could be the basis for studies with larger animals and may help bridge the gap between
the basic understanding of pathophysiologic processes in animal models towards a practical clinical application in liver transplantation" [57]. The findings are especially applicable
in living donor liver transplantation, for which small or margin donor livers were used
for transplantation. Much more pronounced oxidant stress, a higher rate of graft failure,
and retarded graft growth are found in small size liver transplantation than OLT [54, 58].
The margin grafts with small size or steatosis and fibrotic deposition are often used for
transplantation in clinics due to severe shortage of donor organs.

# 6. Challenges in scaling-up and moving towards clinical applications

Our preclinical studies were performed in mice, and there are certainly a number of issues to face when this anti-oxidant gene therapy approach is considered to be evaluated in middle or large size animals such as rabbits, dogs, monkeys or pigs. The first issue is to scale-up, which includes the plasmid DNA generation, synthesis of PCL in a quantity, and formulation of PLNP at a volume sufficient enough for the use in large animals. More challenges exist regarding how to stimulate liver cells to proliferate in large animals and deliver polyplexes locally to the liver. Using a catheter through the femoral vein or jugular vein for retrograde administration into hepatic vein or passing into the portal vein for administration similar to the transjugular intrahepatic portosystemic shunt (TIPS) procedure, which is used to lower portal hypertension in cirrhotic patients, should be feasible in large animals when angiography and the administration are performed by an experienced specialist with the availability of angiographic devices. The latter method was used to administer adenoviral vector in baboons [59]. One trial of plasmid DNA injection into the hepatic vein by blocking the hepatic vein out-flow with an inflated balloon achieved high gene expression levels in selected pig liver lobes [30]. Safety concerns include amount of polyplexes to be administrated locally and the effects of the plasmid DNA, PLNP and polyplexes on the liver as well as systematically. LNP-mediated gene transfer is usually transient; therefore, there will be less concern for long-term effects of the transgene products on the host. However, immune reaction to human gene products in animals may occur if the transgene products are produced at sustained levels for a long period of time. It is preventable by administration of immunosuppressive agents, such as FK506. Moreover, innate immunity to plasmid DNA with bacterial unmethylated CG dinucleotide (CpG) can be eliminated by using CpG-free plasmid [60].

An additional concern is to establish a liver injury model to evaluate the effect of anti-oxidant gene transfer by PLNP in large animals. For pigs, exposure to a loading dose of 0.25 g/kg, maintaining the blood concentration of acetaminophen at 350-450 mg/dl, and adapting enteric maintenance dose of 1,000-3,000 mg/hour resulted in the onset of acute liver failure (prothrombin time value <30%) within 32±4.4 hours, and further mortality in 15.8±2.4 hours [61]. A large dose of acetaminophen intake causes significant oxidant stress and acute liver injury due to its metabolism and generation of an interactive metabolite, n-acetyl-p-benzoquinone imine (NAPQI), which binds to the cytoplasmic membrane, leads to lipid peroxidation, depletion of antioxidants, such as glutathione, and results in hepatic injury. Not only will the delivery of antioxidant genes with PLNP in a pig model of liver injury assess the therapeutic efficacy, but also take advantage of a regenerative response to the injury for high transgene expression. Alternatively, small size graft liver transplantation (SSGLT) at ≤50% graft volume could be performed in rabbits or pigs to mimic living donor liver transplantation in humans. Significant oxidant stress-associated injury and regenerative response in the small size grafts will be the best fit for the high transgene expression and ROS scavenging property of the gene product. Therefore, SSGLT may be considered to be a valuable model for evaluating the feasibility and efficacy of anti-oxidant gene transfer for small-for-size-associated graft failure in a transplant setting.

In summary, moving promising PLNP-mediated antioxidant gene transfer from small animals to large animals may face more challenges than discussed above, and it is even more challenging when further considering for clinical use, in terms of safety concern and administrative approval. Fig. 3 provides a schematic illustration of the roadmap from bench to bedsides of a potential biological therapy. The reality is that with limited funding opportunities from governmental or private agencies, to cope with multi-facet challenges at a large scale, it is less likely to reach the final goal in a short term. Attracting financial investments and taking advantages of cutting-edging technologies and vast resources from biopharmaceutical companies may advance this process in a fast pace. In this context, the net benefits would be the early clinical application of this promising antioxidant gene transfer in patients with critical needs and the financial return from the investment. We would foresee such a movement occurring in the near future.

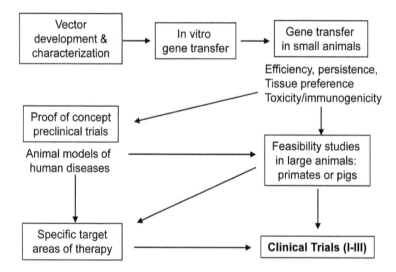

**Figure 3. Translation roadmap of a potential gene therapy platform from bench to bedside.** This illustration summarizes the major steps in moving a potential gene transfer approach from laboratory research to clinical trials. The actual actions could be more complicated than described. However, for the guarantee of patient safety, each new therapeutic agent must be well characterized, and evaluated in preclinical settings, and then move to large animals for feasibility assessment. The balance between therapeutic benefits and potential risks of an innovative therapy platform always leans on the patient safety as the first priority.

## 7. Conclusion and prospectives

Non-viral vector-mediated gene transfer has less concern in terms of integration-associated long-term transgene expression and insertion-induced mutation. In general, non-viral vector elicits minimal immune responses in contrast to adenoviral vectors [17]. However, non-viral vectors, such as lipid nanoparticles (LNPs) possess their own drawbacks when they are considered for *in vivo* use. One prominent issue is the interaction of cationic LNPs with serum protein and blood cells, and this causes a series of issues, such as instability of the lipoplexes or polyplexes and adverse effects to the host, including non-preferential distribution, embolism of the aggregates of lipoplex-protein or blood cells, and inflammatory responses. For these reasons, many gene transfer agents are very effective in cell culture; whereas they have less applicability *in vivo*. Up to date, only a few formulations of cationic LNPs have proved to be effective and safe in animals and have reached the stage of clinical trials, such as DO-TAP-Chol and DC-Chol. Our PLNP formulation has a superior stability profile, and displayed much less reactivity to serum proteins and blood cells when compared to other commercially available formulations. At the same time, it has proved to be the most effective liver-based gene transfer agent [6]. Two preclinical trials with different models of oxidant-stress-associated liver injury have demonstrated the effectiveness of the anti-oxidant gene delivery in the liver, and the efficacy of the gene delivery in minimizing oxidant-stress, attenuating liver cell death, and improving liver histology [48, 49]. Further efforts have been made to move this promising PLNP-mediated anti-oxidant gene transfer technology from bench to bedside. The strategies in pushing this movement towards clinical trials include: 1) Scaling-up of the polycationic lipid production and generation of PLNPs; 2) Generation of specific antioxidant gene plasmids in a GMP facility at the standard for clinical use; 3) Establishing large animal models for safety and efficacy assessment; and 4) Preparation for obtaining administrative approval of clinical application. Although the clinical translation of this potential technology will need tremendous efforts, we anticipate that this technology will eventually reach to patients with critical needs as a novel therapy. Potential indications which may benefit from this therapy range from alcohol or drug toxicity to living donor liver transplantation with a margin graft. This technology is also applicable in oxidant stress-associated disorders in other systems, such as ischemic cardiac, pulmonary, brain or renal damage, etc. [17]. With the combination of our extensive expertise in drug and gene delivery, advanced knowledge and skills in liver injury, fibrosis, transplant and cancer research and practice, in addition to the engine of financial investment from various sources, such as venture capital and governmental support in entrepreneurship, we are optimistic to foresee the benefits of this technology in indicated patients in a near future. Nevertheless, the road to reach this goal will not be smooth, and various challenges demand powerful solutions.

# Acknowledgements

The studies presented in the chapter were supported by the UC Davis Health System Award, American Liver Foundation Liver Scholar Award, UC Davis Technology Transfer Award, and the National Institute of Diabetes, Digestive and Kidney Diseases (DK069939) to JW. The commercialization and translation to clinical application of this technology is supported by the Nanjing Municipal Innovative Technology Award (321 Plan). Yahan Fan is the recipient of China Scholarship Council Award (201207610003).

## Abbreviations used in the chapter

ASGP-R = asialoglycoprotein receptor; DOTAP = (dioleoyloxy)-3-(trimethylamonio) propane; DOPE = L-a dioleoyl phosphatidylethanolamine; EC-SOD = extracellular superoxide dismutase; HCC = hepatocellular carcinoma; LDLT = Living donor liver transplantation; LNP = lipid nanoparticles; OLT = orthotopic liver transplantation; PEG = polyethylene glycol; PLNP = polylipid nanoparticles; polyplex = PLNP-plasmid DNA complex; RES = reticuloendothelial system.

## Author details

Yahan Fan[1,2*] and Jian Wu[1]

*Address all correspondence to: jdwu@ucdavis.edu.

1 Dept. of Internal Medicine, Division of Gastroenterology & Hepatology, University of California, Davis Medical Center, Sacramento, CA, USA

2 Dept. of Internal Medicine, Division of Gastroenterology, Xinqiao Hospital, The Third Military Medical University, Chongqin, P. R. China

## References

[1] Wu J, Zern MA. Modification of liposomes for liver targeting. J Hepatol 1996;24:757-763.

[2] Wu J, Wu GY, Zern MA. The prospects of hepatic drug delivery and gene therapy. Expert Opin Investig Drugs 1998;7:1795-1817.

[3] Du SL, Pan H, Lu WY, Wang J, Wu J, Wang JY. Cyclic Arg-Gly-Asp peptide-labeled liposomes for targeting drug therapy of hepatic fibrosis in rats. J Pharmacol Exp Ther 2007;322:560-568.

[4] Wu J, Liu P, Zhu JL, Maddukuri S, Zern MA. Increased liver uptake of liposomes and improved targeting efficacy by labeling with asialofetuin in rodents. Hepatology 1998;27:772-778.

[5] Abegunewardene N, Schmidt KH, Vosseler M, Kreitner KF, Schreiber LM, Lehr HA, Gori T, et al. Gene therapy with iNOS enhances regional contractility and reduces delayed contrast enhancement in a model of postischemic congestive heart failure. Clin Hemorheol Microcirc 2011;49:271-278.

[6] Liu L, Zern MA, Lizarzaburu ME, Nantz MH, Wu J. Poly(cationic lipid)-mediated in vivo gene delivery to mouse liver. Gene Ther 2003;10:180-187.

[7] Wu J, Lizarzaburu ME, Kurth MJ, Liu L, Wege H, Zern MA, Nantz MH. Cationic lipid polymerization as a novel approach for constructing new DNA delivery agents. Bioconjug Chem 2001;12:251-257.

[8] Nyunt MT, Dicus CW, Cui YY, Yappert MC, Huser TR, Nantz MH, Wu J. Physico-chemical characterization of polylipid nanoparticles for gene delivery to the liver. Bioconjug Chem 2009;20:2047-2054.

[9] Lu C, Stewart DJ, Lee JJ, Ji L, Ramesh R, Jayachandran G, Nunez MI, et al. Phase I clinical trial of systemically administered TUSC2(FUS1)-nanoparticles mediating functional gene transfer in humans. PLoS One 2012;7:e34833.

[10] Ito I, Ji L, Tanaka F, Saito Y, Gopalan B, Branch CD, Xu K, et al. Liposomal vector mediated delivery of the 3p FUS1 gene demonstrates potent antitumor activity against human lung cancer in vivo. Cancer Gene Ther 2004;11:733-739.

[11] Sakurai F, Nishioka T, Saito H, Baba T, Okuda A, Matsumoto O, Taga T, et al. Interaction between DNA-cationic liposome complexes and erythrocytes is an important factor in systemic gene transfer via the intravenous route in mice: the role of the neutral helper lipid. Gene Ther 2001;8:677-686.

[12] Fumoto S, Kawakami S, Shigeta K, Higuchi Y, Yamashita F, Hashida M. Interaction with blood components plays a crucial role in asialoglycoprotein receptor-mediated in vivo gene transfer by galactosylated lipoplex. J Pharmacol Exp Ther 2005;315:484-493.

[13] Fumoto S, Kawakami S, Ito Y, Shigeta K, Yamashita F, Hashida M. Enhanced hepatocyte-selective in vivo gene expression by stabilized galactosylated liposome/plasmid DNA complex using sodium chloride for complex formation. Mol Ther 2004;10:719-729.

[14] Liu Y, Mounkes LC, Liggitt HD, Brown CS, Solodin I, Heath TD, Debs RJ. Factors influencing the efficiency of cationic liposome-mediated intravenous gene delivery. Nat Biotechnol 1997;15:167-173.

[15] Schleh C, Rothen-Rutishauser B, Kreyling WG. The influence of pulmonary surfactant on nanoparticulate drug delivery systems. Eur J Pharm Biopharm 2011;77:350-352.

[16] Ramesh R, Ito I, Saito Y, Wu Z, Mhashikar AM, Wilson DR, Branch CD, et al. Local and systemic inhibition of lung tumor growth after nanoparticle-mediated mda-7/IL-24 gene delivery. DNA Cell Biol 2004;23:850-857.

[17] Wu J, Hecker JG, Chiamvimonvat N. Antioxidant enzyme gene transfer for ischemic diseases. Adv Drug Deliv Rev 2009;61:351-363.

[18] Wei M, Xu Y, Zou Q, Tu L, Tang C, Xu T, Deng L, et al. Hepatocellular carcinoma targeting effect of PEGylated liposomes modified with lactoferrin. Eur J Pharm Sci 2012;46:131-141.

[19] Zheng S, Chang S, Lu J, Chen Z, Xie L, Nie Y, He B, et al. Characterization of 9-nitro-camptothecin liposomes: anticancer properties and mechanisms on hepatocellular carcinoma in vitro and in vivo. PLoS One 2011;6:e21064.

[20] Khalil IA, Hayashi Y, Mizuno R, Harashima H. Octaarginine- and pH sensitive fuso-genic peptide-modified nanoparticles for liver gene delivery. J Control Release 2011;156:374-380.

[21] Karmali PP, Chaudhuri A. Cationic liposomes as non-viral carriers of gene medi-cines: resolved issues, open questions, and future promises. Med Res Rev 2007;27:696-722.

[22] Al-Jamal WT, Kostarelos K. Liposomes: from a clinically established drug delivery system to a nanoparticle platform for theranostic nanomedicine. Acc Chem Res 2011;44:1094-1104.

[23] Li Y, Zhu Y, Xia K, Sheng R, Jia L, Hou X, Xu Y, et al. Dendritic poly(L-lysine)-b-Poly(L-lactide)-b-dendritic poly(L-lysine) amphiphilic gene delivery vectors: roles of PLL dendritic generation and enhanced transgene efficacies via termini modification. Biomacromolecules 2009;10:2284-2293.

[24] Byeon JH, Kim HK, Roberts JT. Monodisperse Poly(lactide-co-glycolic acid)-Based Nanocarriers for Gene Transfection. Macromol Rapid Commun 2012; 23:1821-1825.

[25] Nogueira N, Conde O, Minones M, Trillo JM, Minones J, Jr. Characterization of poly(2-hydroxyethyl methacrylate) (PHEMA) contact lens using the Langmuir mon-olayer technique. J Colloid Interface Sci 2012;385:202-210.

[26] So H, Lee J, Han SY, Oh HB. MALDI In-Source Decay Mass Spectrometry of Polya-midoamine Dendrimers. J Am Soc Mass Spectrometry 2012:DOI: 10.1007/s13361-13012-10445-13364.

[27] Poelstra K, Prakash J, Beljaars L. Drug targeting to the diseased liver. J Control Re-lease 2012;161:188-197.

[28] Wu J, Nantz MH, Zern MA. Targeting hepatocytes for drug and gene delivery: emerging novel approaches and applications. Front Biosci 2002;7:d717-725.

[29] Alino SF, Benet M, Dasi F, Crespo J. Asialofetuin liposomes for receptor-mediated gene transfer into hepatic cells. Methods Enzymol 2003;373:399-421.

[30] Alino SF, Herrero MJ, Noguera I, Dasi F, Sanchez M. Pig liver gene therapy by nonin-vasive interventionist catheterism. Gene Ther 2007;14:334-343.

[31] Li Y, Huang G, Diakur J, Wiebe LI. Targeted delivery of macromolecular drugs: asia-loglycoprotein receptor (ASGPR) expression by selected hepatoma cell lines used in antiviral drug development. Curr Drug Deliv 2008;5:299-302.

[32] Chen X, Lingala S, Khoobyari S, Nolta J, Zern MA, Wu J. Epithelial mesenchymal transition and hedgehog signaling activation are associated with chemoresistance and invasion of hepatoma subpopulations. J Hepatol 2011;55:838-845.

[33]  Hyodo I, Mizuno M, Yamada G, Tsuji T. Distribution of asialoglycoprotein receptor in human hepatocellular carcinoma. Liver 1993;13:80-85.

[34]  Sawamura T, Nakada H, Hazama H, Shiozaki Y, Sameshima Y, Tashiro Y. Hyperasialoglycoproteinemia in patients with chronic liver diseases and/or liver cell carcinoma. Asialoglycoprotein receptor in cirrhosis and liver cell carcinoma. Gastroenterology 1984;87:1217-1221.

[35]  Dorasamy S, Narainpersad N, Singh M, Ariatti M. Novel targeted liposomes deliver siRNA to hepatocellular carcinoma cells in vitro. Chem Biol Drug Des 2012:10.1111/j. 1747-0285.2012.01446.x.

[36]  Feng M, Cai Q, Shi X, Huang H, Zhou P, Guo X. Recombinant high-density lipoprotein complex as a targeting system of nosiheptide to liver cells. J Drug Targeting 2008;16:502-508.

[37]  Akinc A, Querbes W, De S, Qin J, Frank-Kamenetsky M, Jayaprakash KN, Jayaraman M, et al. Targeted delivery of RNAi therapeutics with endogenous and exogenous ligand-based mechanisms. Mol Ther 2010;18:1357-1364.

[38]  Wu J, Zern MA. Hepatic stellate cells: a target for the treatment of liver fibrosis. J Gastroenterol 2000;35:665-672.

[39]  Beljaars L, Molema G, Weert B, Bonnema H, Olinga P, Groothuis GM, Meijer DK, et al. Albumin modified with mannose 6-phosphate: A potential carrier for selective delivery of antifibrotic drugs to rat and human hepatic stellate cells. Hepatology 1999;29:1486-1493.

[40]  Li F, Li QH, Wang JY, Zhan CY, Xie C, Lu WY. Effects of interferon-gamma liposomes targeted to platelet-derived growth factor receptor-beta on hepatic fibrosis in rats. J Control Release 2012;159:261-270.

[41]  Beljaars L, Olinga P, Molema G, de Bleser P, Geerts A, Groothuis GM, Meijer DK, et al. Characteristics of the hepatic stellate cell-selective carrier mannose 6-phosphate modified albumin (M6P(28)-HSA). Liver 2001;21:320-328.

[42]  Li F, Song Z, Li Q, Wu J, Wang J, Xie C, Tu C, et al. Molecular imaging of hepatic stellate cell activity by visualization of hepatic integrin alphavbeta3 expression with SPECT in rat. Hepatology 2011;54:1020-1030.

[43]  Sato Y, Murase K, Kato J, Kobune M, Sato T, Kawano Y, Takimoto R, et al. Resolution of liver cirrhosis using vitamin A-coupled liposomes to deliver siRNA against a collagen-specific chaperone. Nat Biotechnol 2008;26:431-442.

[44]  Yen RD, Zern MA, Wu J. Molecular therapy for hepatic fibrosis. Hauppauge, NY.: Nova Science Publishers, 2006: 1-23.

[45]  Nishikawa M, Huang L. Nonviral vectors in the new millennium: delivery barriers in gene transfer. Hum Gene Ther 2001;12:861-870.

[46] Diez S, Navarro G, de ICT. In vivo targeted gene delivery by cationic nanoparticles for treatment of hepatocellular carcinoma. J Gene Med 2009;11:38-45.

[47] Li S, Rizzo MA, Bhattacharya S, Huang L. Characterization of cationic lipid-prota-mine-DNA (LPD) complexes for intravenous gene delivery. Gene Ther 1998;5:930-937.

[48] Wu J, Liu L, Yen RD, Catana A, Nantz MH, Zern MA. Liposome-mediated extracel-lular superoxide dismutase gene delivery protects against acute liver injury in mice. Hepatology 2004;40:195-204.

[49] He SQ, Zhang YH, Venugopal SK, Dicus CW, Perez RV, Ramsamooj R, Nantz MH, et al. Delivery of antioxidative enzyme genes protects against ischemia/reperfusion-in-duced liver injury in mice. Liver Transpl 2006;12:1869-1879.

[50] Wu J, Danielsson A, Zern MA. Toxicity of hepatotoxins: new insights into mecha-nisms and therapy. Expert Opin Investig Drugs 1999;8:585-607.

[51] Wu J, Karlsson K, Danielsson A. Effects of vitamins E, C and catalase on bromoben-zene- and hydrogen peroxide-induced intracellular oxidation and DNA single-strand breakage in Hep G2 cells. J Hepatol 1997;26:669-677.

[52] Wu J, Karlsson K, Danielsson A. Protective effects of trolox C, vitamin C, and cata-lase on bromobenzene-induced damage to rat hepatocytes. Scand J Gastroenterol 1996;31:797-803.

[53] Wu J, Soderbergh H, Karlsson K, Danielsson A. Protective effect of S-adenosyl-L-me-thionine on bromobenzene- and D-galactosamine-induced toxicity to isolated rat hepatocytes. Hepatology 1996;23:359-365.

[54] Cui Y-Y, Qian J-M, Yao A-H, Ma Z-Y, Qian X-F, Zha X-M, Zhao Y, et al. SOD mimetic improves the function, growth, and survival of small-size liver grafts after transplan-tation in rats. Transplantation 2012; 94:687-694.

[55] Qian JM, Zhang H, Wu XF, Li GQ, Chen XP, Wu J. Improvement of recipient survival after small size graft liver transplantation in rats with preischemic manipulation or administering antisense against nuclear factor-kappaB. Transplant Int 2007;20:784-789.

[56] Liu PG, He SQ, Zhang YH, Wu J. Protective effects of apocynin and allopurinol on ischemia/reperfusion-induced liver injury in mice. World J Gastroenterol 2008;14:2832-2837.

[57] Luedde T, Trautwein C. The role of oxidative stress and antioxidant treatment in liv-er surgery and transplantation. Liver Transpl 2006;12:1733-1735.

[58] Cerullo V, Seiler MP, Mane V, Brunetti-Pierri N, Clarke C, Bertin TK, Rodgers JR, et al. Toll-like receptor 9 triggers an innate immune response to helper-dependent ade-noviral vectors. Mol Ther 2007;15:378-385.

[59]  Brunetti-Pierri N, Stapleton GE, Palmer DJ, Zuo Y, Mane VP, Finegold MJ, Beaudet AL, et al. Pseudo-hydrodynamic delivery of helper-dependent adenoviral vectors into non-human primates for liver-directed gene therapy. Mol Ther 2007;15:732-740.

[60]  Hyde SC, Pringle IA, Abdullah S, Lawton AE, Davies LA, Varathalingam A, Nunez-Alonso G, et al. CpG-free plasmids confer reduced inflammation and sustained pulmonary gene expression. Nat Biotechnol 2008;26:549-551.

[61]  Thiel C, Thiel K, Etspueler A, Morgalla MH, Rubitschek S, Schmid S, Steurer W, et al. A reproducible porcine model of acute liver failure induced by intrajejunal acetaminophen administration. Eur Surg Res 2011;46:118-126.

# Permissions

The contributors of this book come from diverse backgrounds, making this book a truly international effort. This book will bring forth new frontiers with its revolutionizing research information and detailed analysis of the nascent developments around the world.

We would like to thank Francisco Martín Molina, for lending his expertise to make the book truly unique. He has played a crucial role in the development of this book. Without his invaluable contribution this book wouldn't have been possible. He has made vital efforts to compile up to date information on the varied aspects of this subject to make this book a valuable addition to the collection of many professionals and students.

This book was conceptualized with the vision of imparting up-to-date information and advanced data in this field. To ensure the same, a matchless editorial board was set up. Every individual on the board went through rigorous rounds of assessment to prove their worth. After which they invested a large part of their time researching and compiling the most relevant data for our readers. Conferences and sessions were held from time to time between the editorial board and the contributing authors to present the data in the most comprehensible form. The editorial team has worked tirelessly to provide valuable and valid information to help people across the globe.

Every chapter published in this book has been scrutinized by our experts. Their significance has been extensively debated. The topics covered herein carry significant findings which will fuel the growth of the discipline. They may even be implemented as practical applications or may be referred to as a beginning point for another development. Chapters in this book were first published by InTech; hereby published with permission under the Creative Commons Attribution License or equivalent.

The editorial board has been involved in producing this book since its inception. They have spent rigorous hours researching and exploring the diverse topics which have resulted in the successful publishing of this book. They have passed on their knowledge of decades through this book. To expedite this challenging task, the publisher supported the team at every step. A small team of assistant editors was also appointed to further simplify the editing procedure and attain best results for the readers.

Our editorial team has been hand-picked from every corner of the world. Their multi-ethnicity adds dynamic inputs to the discussions which result in innovative outcomes. These outcomes are then further discussed with the researchers and contributors who give their valuable feedback and opinion regarding the same. The feedback is then collaborated with the researches and they are edited in a comprehensive manner to aid the understanding of the subject.

Apart from the editorial board, the designing team has also invested a significant amount of their time in understanding the subject and creating the most relevant covers. They scrutinized every image to scout for the most suitable representation of the subject and create an appropriate cover for the book.

The publishing team has been involved in this book since its early stages. They were actively engaged in every process, be it collecting the data, connecting with the contributors or procuring relevant information. The team has been an ardent support to the editorial, designing and production team. Their endless efforts to recruit the best for this project, has resulted in the accomplishment of this book. They are a veteran in the field of academics and their pool of knowledge is as vast as their experience in printing. Their expertise and guidance has proved useful at every step. Their uncompromising quality standards have made this book an exceptional effort. Their encouragement from time to time has been an inspiration for everyone.

The publisher and the editorial board hope that this book will prove to be a valuable piece of knowledge for researchers, students, practitioners and scholars across the globe.

# List of Contributors

Alicia Rodríguez Gascón, Ana del Pozo-Rodríguez and María Ángeles Solinís
Pharmacokinetics, Nanotechnology and Gene Therapy Group, Faculty of Phamacy, University of the Basque Country UPV/EHU, Spain

Oleg E. Tolmachov
St. Mary's University College, Twickenham, UK

Tatiana Subkhankulova and Tanya Tolmachova
National Heart and Lung Institute, Imperial College London, London, UK

David Morrissey, Sara A. Collins, Simon Rajenderan, Garrett Casey, Gerald C. O'Sullivan and Mark Tangney
Cork Cancer Research Centre, Mercy University Hospital and Leslie C. Quick Jnr. Laboratory, University College Cork, Cork, Ireland

Aurore Burgain-Chain and Daniel Scherman
Unit of Chemical and Genetic Pharmacology and of Bioimaging, CNRS Paris, Université Paris Descartes, Chimie Paris Tech, Paris-Sorbonne PRES, France

Abdelkader A. Metwally
Department of Pharmacy and Pharmacology, University of Bath, Bath BA2 7AY, UK
Department of Pharmaceutics and Industrial Pharmacy, Faculty of Pharmacy, Ain Shams University, Abbasya, Cairo, Egypt

Ian S. Blagbrough
Department of Pharmacy and Pharmacology, University of Bath, Bath BA2 7AY, UK

Shengnan Xiang and Xiaoling Zhang
The Key Laboratory of Stem Cell Biology, Institute of Health Sciences, Shanghai Jiao Tong University School of Medicine (SJTUSM) & Shanghai Institutes for Biological Sciences (SIBS), Chinese Academy of Sciences (CAS), Shanghai, China

Yahan Fan
Dept. of Internal Medicine, Division of Gastroenterology & Hepatology, University of California, Davis Medical Center, Sacramento, CA, USA
Dept. of Internal Medicine, Division of Gastroenterology, Xinqiao Hospital, The Third Military Medical University, Chongqin, P. R. China

Jian Wu
Dept. of Internal Medicine, Division of Gastroenterology & Hepatology, University of California, Davis Medical Center, Sacramento, CA, USA